HOMOEOPATHY FOR PHYSICIANS

A Practical Introduction to Prescribing

by
Colin B. Lessell

M.B., B.S.(Lond.), B.D.S.(Lond.), M.R.C.S.(Eng.), L.R.C.P.(Lond.)

THORSONS PUBLISHERS LIMITED
Wellingborough, Northamptonshire

First published 1983

British Library Cataloguing in Publication Data

Lessell, Colin B.
  Homoeopathy for physicians.
  1. Pharmacopoeias, Homoeopathic
  I. Title
  615.5'32   RX675
  ISBN 0-7225-0798-4

Printed and bound in Great Britain

HOMEOPATHY FOR PHYSICIANS

A straightforward guide to the principles of homeopathy, and clearly laid down guidelines for practitioners for their application in the treatment of acute and chronic disease.

Contents

	Page
Introduction	7

PART ONE: The Principles of Homoeopathy and their
Application to the Treatment of Acute Disease

1. Dr Samuel Hahnemann and the Law of Similars	9
2. The Preparation of Remedies, and Scales of Dilution	11
3. The Administration of Remedies and their Storage	15
4. An Initial Exercise in Practical Prescribing	18
5. The Similimum	21
6. Basic Remedies	23
7. Home Remedy Kits	28
8. Prescribing in Acute Disease	33
9. Fever and Acute Otitis Media	35
10. Colds, Influenza and Respiratory Infection	37
11. The Ill-effects of Antibiotics	39
12. Specific Infectious Fevers of Childhood	40
13. Homoeopathic Preventative Medicine	42
14. Sequential, Concurrent and Alternate Prescribing	44
15. Sudden Collapse	47
16. Infective Disease of the Skin	48
17. Acute Orthopaedic Problems	49
18. Acute Abdominal Complaints	50
19. Pregnancy and Lactation	51
20. Works of Reference	53
21. Test Paper	58

PART TWO: The Theory and Treatment of the Chronic
Diseases

22. The Nature of Chronic Disease	61
23. Fundamental Disease: Genetic and Cellular	63
24. Modifying Factors: Environment, Nutrition and Infection	68
25. The Concept of Cure	72
26. The Complexity of Chronic Disease	75
27. A Sensible Basic Diet	77
28. Constipation	80

29. Indigestion   81
30. Diet in Arthritis   83
31. Hypoglycaemia   84
32. The Grape Cure   87
33. Veganism and Vegetarianism   89
34. Aluminium Sensitivity   90
35. Food Allergy   92
36. Dietetic Supplements   99
37. Constitutional and Pathological Prescribing   102
38. General Constitutional Prescribing   109
39. Major General Constitutional Remedies   116
40. The Selection of Potency   124
41. Practical Aspects of General Constitutional
    Prescribing, and the Law of Cure   127
42. Are Drugs and Homoeopathic Remedies Compatible?   136
43. Antimiasmatic Remedies   138
44. Pathological Remedies   145
45. Final Summary   152
46. Test Paper   155
    Useful Addresses   157
    Index   158

Introduction

This book is dedicated to the physician who wishes to acquire a working knowledge of homoeopathy. There is, after all, a rapidly growing interest amongst both the members of our ancient profession and our patients in what has come to be termed 'wholistic medicine', of which homoeopathy is very much a part. Wholistic medicine is a synthesis of those healing disciplines that recognize the intimate union in each individual of spirit, mind and body, and the relationships of that individual with the immediate environment, fellow beings, and the cosmos in general. For many physicians, and our numbers are multiplying, homoeopathy is the link between their orthodox training and these wholistic concepts. The founder of homoeopathy was himself a conventionally trained physician.

Do not fear being labelled a reactionary, when your conscience determines that you must discover a greater view of the healing arts. You must practise medicine according to the dictates of your own conscience. It is not for me, therefore, to implore you to study the homoeopathic method, but rather to assume that you travel this path of your own accord, and that you seek a guide for the journey. Unlike your conscience, the guide cannot dictate. He can merely advise. One day, the traveller might himself become the guide for another.

It has been my decision, therefore, to adopt an informal approach to this work. It is comprised of a number of dialogues, rather than chapters. I would like you to feel that I am talking to you directly. I, in turn, must attempt to anticipate some of your questions, and answer them to the best of my ability. Consider this book as a pleasant conversation between one colleague and another. Whether we will have simply passed the time of day, or otherwise, it will be for you to say.

My main objective is to give you enough information to begin prescribing homoeopathic remedies; for clinical success is the best means of demonstrating the efficacy of any method. The proof of any theoretical pudding must be in the empirical eating. But first we must take a little time to understand how our pudding is made.

PART ONE

The Principles of Homoeopathy and their Application to the Treatment of Acute Disease

1.

Dr Samuel Hahnemann and the Law of Similars

Homoeopathy is that school of medicine founded by Dr Christian Frederick Samuel Hahnemann, who was born at Meissen in Germany in 1755, and died in Paris in 1843. The experimental and practical foundation studies for homoeopathy were carried out between the years 1790 and 1810, culminating in the publication of Hahnemann's first major work, *The Organon*.

Hahnemann's fundamental propositions, peculiar to homoeopathy, may be expressed thus:

1. That the action of drugs is demonstrable by observing the signs (objective symptoms), symptoms (subjective symptoms), and pathological changes that occur when they are administered to *healthy* human subjects.

2. That the action of drugs in the *healthy* constitutes their therapeutic potential with respect to the sick.

3. That a *similarity* between the disease process in a particular individual, and the known effects of a particular drug in the healthy will lead to its successful application in the treatment of that diseased individual.

These propositions are succinctly implied in the so-called *Law of Similars,* which is the foundation of all medicinal homoeopathic practice. *Similia similibus curentur:* 'Let likes be treated with likes'.

The Law of Similars is a natural law, rather like the laws of mechanics. It defines a simple method by which drugs may be selected for the treatment of patients. The drug *Cinchona officinalis* (Peruvian bark), containing quinine, will produce malaria-like symptoms when repeatedly administered to healthy *human* volunteers. Its use, therefore, in the treatment of patients with malaria, is in accordance with the Law of Similars. The orthodox methods of vaccination, immunization, and allergen desensitization are similarly in accord with the homoeopathic law. The term *homoeopathy* is, in fact, derived from the Greek, meaning 'like suffering'. Orthodox medicine is termed *allopathy*.

Now, at this juncture, you might say: 'All very interesting, but so what?' The Law of Similars appears on the surface to be no more than a novel way of selecting drugs to match the patient. Yet, there is far more to it. Let us examine Hahnemann's dosage in the period 1798-1799, as given to us by Dr Richard Hughes, in order to see what I mean.

In 1798 we find Hahnemann speaking of doses such as: *Ignatia,* 2 or 3 grains (1 grain = 65mg); *Opium,* $\frac{1}{2}$ grain; *Camphor,* 30 or 40 grains; *Ledum,* 6 to 7 grains; *Cinchona,* 1 drachm (3.9g). These are obvious material dosages of drugs.

In 1799, however, we find a considerable change in prescribing: *Opium,* one five-millionth of a grain; *Belladonna,* one 432,000th part of a grain, and so on. An enormous reduction in dosage!

Hahnemann had discovered that the application of drugs *in accordance with the Law of Similars* enabled those drugs to be applied in the most minute quantities and still maintain therapeutic efficacy.

Genius or madman? Had Hahnemann discovered a means of preserving pharmacological activity, whilst rejecting biochemical toxicity? Well, madman he was not! As you will discover, homoeopathic remedies are not simple extreme dilutions. They are something more, and they *are* pharmacologically active.

By utilizing the Law of Similars, drugs may be applied to the sick in a manner that rids us of the problems of direct toxicity.

2.

The Preparation of Remedies, and Scales of Dilution

In the early days of homoeopathy the physician would have been expected to prepare his own medicinal remedies. Nowadays, and laudably for the busy practitioner, we may obtain our remedies from properly trained homoeopathic pharmacists; but it still behoves us to understand the methods by which they are produced. We prefer to use the term *remedies* for our preparations, to distinguish them from the crude drugs of origin.

There are three essential processes involved in the preparation of remedies: *serial dilution, succussion,* and *trituration.* Dilution is the means by which we reduce the toxicity of the original crude drug. Serial dilution means that each dilution is prepared from the dilution that immediately precedes it. Succussion and trituration are the methods by which mechanical energy is delivered to our preparations in order to imprint the pharmacological message of the original drug upon *the molecules of diluent.*

From the pharmaceutical point of view, there are two main classes of original substance: *soluble,* and *insoluble.* In the class of soluble substances, mother tinctures (alcoholic extractions) of plant material are used with great frequency. The symbol $\emptyset$ is used to denote the mother tincture of any soluble substance. For soluble substances, the diluent applied is alcohol-water. At each stage of serial dilution, violent agitation is carried out, either by hand or machine, and this is what we mean by *succussion.*

Insoluble original substances, such as flint (*Silicea*), are prepared differently in the initial stages. Here the diluent is lactose ('sac. lac.'). The physical process applied at each dilution is *trituration*: prolonged grinding with mortar and pestle, or similar mechanical device. Once a dilution in excess of $1/10^6$ has been attained, the originally insoluble substance can be colloidally dispersed in alcohol-water diluent. Thereafter, the material is treated as for soluble substances.

There are two major scales of serial dilution: the centesimal or 'c' scale, and the decimal or 'x' scale. The centesimal scale involves serial dilutions of 1/100. The decimal scale involves serial dilutions of 1/10. As I have stated, according to the solubility of the drug, so the appropriate method of either succussion or trituration *must* be applied at each stage of dilution.

Here are the mathematics in tabular form:

Potency	No. episodes of trituration/succussion	Dilution
(∅	0	0)
1c	1	1/100
1x	1	1/10
6x	6	$1/10^6$
6c	6	$1/10^{12}$
12x	12	$1/10^{12}$
30c	30	$1/10^{60}$
200c	200	$1/10^{400}$
1M (=1000c)	1000	$1/10^{2000}$
10M (=10000c)	10000	$1/10^{20000}$
CM (=100000c)	100000	$1/10^{200000}$

The following points are worthy of note:

1. The term *potency* refers to any dilution that has been either succussed or triturated. This serves to distinguish it from a simple dilution. Similarly, the process of remedy preparation is termed *potentization*.

2. When prescribing remedies, the potency suffix should always be stated, e.g. *Arsenicum album* 30c. Since the centesimal scale is the one more commonly used in professional practice, many physicians and pharmacists tend to drop the 'c'. Hence, *Arsenicum album* 30 = *Arsenicum album* 30c. By contrast, the 'x' notation is used consistently where the decimal scale is intended.

3. The potency symbol M is an abbreviation for 1000c. Hence, *Zincum metallicum* 50M = *Zincum metallicum* 50000c.

4. Occasionally you will come across Continental potencies, usually French or German in origin. Their abbreviations are different: cH = c, and D = x. Hence, 30cH = 30c, and D12 = 12x.

5. You will have observed that the potencies 6c and 12x both represent a dilution factor of $1/10^{12}$. They differ, however, in

that the x potency has undergone twelve episodes of succussion/ trituration, whilst the c potency has only undergone six episodes. Their therapeutic potentials are, therefore, by no means identical. 12x is more potent than 6c.

6. At a dilution of $1/10^{24}$, corresponding to potencies of 12c or 24x, Avogadro's limit has been reached, beyond which there are theoretically no molecules of original substance left in the preparation. However, it is clinically and experimentally demonstrable that such potencies are still pharmacologically active. Moreover, not only are they simply pharmacologically active, but they preserve the therapeutic potential of the original drug in a most remarkable manner. It is held that the methods of potentization cause the pharmacological message of the original drug to be impressed, so to speak, on the water molecules of the diluent (there will be water molecules present in large quantity even in trituration). This may involve a polymerization or electromagnetic effect. It is the solvent, therefore, that carries the pharmacological message from one serial dilution to the next. Certainly, if remedial preparations are allowed to desiccate, they become therapeutically inactive.

7. Speaking generally, the higher the potency, the more potent is the remedy. 200c is considerably more potent than 6c.

8. The most commonly used potencies in practice are: 6x, 6c, 12c, 30c, 200c, 1M, 10M, CM. The use of decimal preparations above 30x is seldom warranted.

9. The dilution factor seems to play a part in the generation of potency. Both 6c and 6x potencies have undergone six episodes of mechanical agitation, yet the 6c potency appears more potent in therapeutic action. The centesimal scale is the 'stronger'.

10. Overtly toxic substances, such as arsenic, are rendered non-toxic by serial dilution, and, therefore, may be used clinically. Whereas *Arsenicum album* 2x still contains residual molecules in significant quantity of original substance, and thus would not be prescribable, a potency 12c is free of original substance, and is frequently used clinically.

11. Essentially pharmacologically inert substances, such as *Lycopodium* (Club-moss spores), can be rendered pharmacologically active by the methods of potentization. In order to ascertain the therapeutic potential of such substances, they must, of necessity, be administered *in potency* to healthy volunteers. In the crude state they are totally devoid of pharmacological action.

Now, chew these points over before we proceed. If they seem a little indigestible at first, take some *Nux vomica* 6 (Poison-nut)! At a dilution of 1/1000000000000, it contains only a negligible quantity of strychnine.

3.

The Administration of Remedies
and their Storage

You now know the basics of remedial preparation. There are three main types of substance available for therapy:
1. Triturations of insoluble substances up to 6x potency.
2. Succussed liquid potencies.
3. Mother tinctures of negligible toxicity.

Triturated material may be administered as powders (usually enclosed in folded paper and often numbered), or may be compressed into flat tablet form. Liquid potencies may be administered as such, or may be used to impregnate inert lactose, which may be in the form of powders, granules, tablets, or spherical pilules. For topical use, the liquid potency may be combined with a bland cream or ointment base. Tinctures are generally given as drops in a little water for oral use. They may be diluted with water to yield lotions, or may be put up as creams or ointments.

Homoeopathic remedies are generally given orally for a systemic action. They are rapidly absorbed by the oral mucosa, and patients are advised to allow them to dissolve either on or under the tongue. Because of their sweet taste, the lactose preparations find great favour with children. The amount of sugar contained in each dose is, however, so small that dental caries or exacerbation of diabetes are not to be considered as risks. Occasionally, a patient may complain that the remedy tastes 'peculiar'. This is generally a good sign, for it only appears to happen when the remedy is well indicated for the patient. An absence of peculiar taste, however, does not mean that the remedy is poorly chosen. It is largely arbitrary whether the remedy for oral use is given as powder, tablet, pilule, or in drop form. In real therapeutic terms, their efficacies are identical. For small children or unconscious patients, however, it is prudent to use either powders or drops, for pills or tablets may be inhaled, with dire consequences. Even if only pilules or tablets are available, they may be readily crushed into a fine powder for safe use.

The matter of dosage requires some discussion.

Homoeopathic remedies *trigger* reactions of the physiology. If the pull on the trigger of a gun is set for 1kg, there is no advantage to be gained with a pull of 10kg, for the gun will fire with no greater force. Enough is enough, so to speak. Thus, we find in clinical practice that one pill, one tablet, an equivalent amount of powder, or one or two drops of liquid potency are adequate in *all age-groups* to fire the physiology. There is no advantage to be gained (except a psychological one) by giving ten tablets simultaneously, or a cupful of drops. It is certainly not harmful to do so, but it is ridiculously wasteful. In order to achieve a greater effect, either a different potency must be administered, or the remedy must be repeated at intervals. Generally, the higher potencies exhibit a more marked and long-lasting effect. Only in the case of certain mother tinctures, of low toxicity and low pharmacological energy (e.g. *Crataegus,* Hawthorn berry), is it sometimes necessary to prescribe as many as five drops as a single dose.

Whereas it is possible to administer remedies by injection, as suppositories, or by inhalation, these methods are seldom, if ever, indicated. The topical use of *Hamamelis virginica* (Witch-hazel) suppositories for haemorrhoids is a notable exception.

Homoeopathic creams, ointments, or lotions, however, may be usefully combined with systemic treatment. *Graphites* 8x (pencil-lead) cream may be found of use in alleviating, though not necessarily curing, cases of weeping eczema. *Calendula* Ø (Marigold) 5% cream is the great healer to be applied to cuts, abrasions, scalds and operative wounds. *Urtica urens* Ø (Stinging-nettle), diluted with sterile water 1/5, is an excellent lotion for burns. *Euphrasia officinalis* Ø (Eyebright) may be diluted to make a lotion suitable for the treatment of conjunctivitis.

Where topical treatment is instituted, the administration of synergistic oral remedies is generally to be recommended.

Because of the delicate nature of homoeopathic remedies, certain precautions should be taken. Patients should be informed not to eat, drink, or clean their teeth within fifteen minutes of taking an oral remedy. Coffee, whether decaffeinated or not, is a great antidote to the action of many, though not all, remedies, and should, therefore, be proscribed during the term of treatment. Remedies should be handled minimally, and should be kept in well-stoppered amber containers. The finest material for these is glass, especially if long term storage is anticipated (over three years). Plastic containers are satisfactory for lesser periods of storage. It must always be remembered that the internal walls of the container are contaminated with the potentized remedy, even if this is invisible to the naked eye. Remedies should thus not be transferred from their container of issue to others that have contained different remedies. Dehydration, or the prolonged exposure to sunlight, destroys potency. Artificial light is of no consequence. Perfumes and other aromatic substances, especially camphor, destroy potency, and must, therefore, be kept away from remedies. Kept in a cool place to avoid dehydration, in well sealed containers, the shelf life of remedies is considerable: ten, twenty, thirty years or more.

4.

An Initial Exercise
in Practical Prescribing

You are now ready to write your first homoeopathic prescriptions. These will serve to 'break the ice' for both you and your patients. It is, in my opinion, most important to do this before we embark on those more complex aspects of prescribing, in order to give encouragement for further study. You can expect a reasonable degree of success with the measures suggested, but remember to review all cases periodically in order to make this assessment. Take a personal interest in what is, or *is not,* happening. Even if it is not feasible for you to see the patient for review, get someone to call you on the telephone about their progress.

To start with, you must obtain for your own dispensary the preparations given below, *before* you commence prescribing. Alternatively, ask your local pharmacist to stock them for your patients. In either event, they are readily available from distributing homoeopathic pharmacies. You will require the following:

Calendula Ø 5% cream, 3 X 35g tubes.

Pilules *Arnica montana* 30c, 3 X 7g bottles.

Euphrasia officinalis Ø, 3 X 5ml dropper bottles.

Pilules *Euphrasia officinalis* 12c, 3 X 7g bottles.

Each 7g bottle contains approximately 60-70 pilules. The pilules will vary slightly in size, but this is of no consequence with regard to dosage. Each pilule, irrespective of size contains more than enough medicament to trigger the healing response.

You now have the potential to prescribe for three patients in each of the three clinical categories that follow:

1. *Simple topical prescribing.* You may select patients suffering from: cuts, abrasions, minor burns, or recent episiotomy incisions. Prescribe: *Calendula* Ø 5% cream, 35g, apply sparingly tid. Observe the results.

2. *Simple systemic prescribing.* You may select patients suffering from: severe traumatic bruising, or sprained ankle. Prescribe: Pilules *Arnica montana* 30c, 7g, i tid, or i every hour if pain or swelling is severe. Observe the results.

Arnica montana (Leopard's bane) is the greatest of all the anti-bruise and anti-sprain remedies. It may be prescribed in other potencies, such as 6c, 12c, 200c, but 30c is probably the commonest. It may also be applied as a lotion, 5 drops of Ø to one fluid ounce (28ml) of water. *Arnica* (we generally drop *montana*) additionally has a reputation for diminishing muscle fatigue following vigorous exercise, and thus is of service in mild lumbago following gardening.

3. *Simple mixed prescribing* (systemic and topical). For this exercise, select patients suffering from uncomplicated acute conjunctivitis. Prescribe: Pilules *Euphrasia* 12c (again it is permissible to omit *officinalis*), 7g, i tid. You must order that they are to be crushed if for a baby. Additionally, *Euphrasia* Ø, 5ml in dropper bottle, 5-10 drops to a fluid ounce (28ml) of water as an eyewash for adults (10 drops may yield an eyewash that is a little too strong for very sensitive eyes, and cause mild stinging; it is better, therefore, to commence with a weaker solution, and gradually increase the strength). For children, have the pharmacist make the appropriate dilution, and issue it in a 10ml rubber pipette bottle so that the parents may instil one or two drops directly into the conjunctival sac. Never allow patients to use a more concentrated solution, since the high alcoholic content of the Ø will burn the eye. The eyewash or drops should be applied three or four times daily. Observe the results. Bottles of prepared eyedrops must be discarded after use.

Remember that all patients taking remedies should be furnished with information regarding how to take them, and look after them. It is most convenient, therefore, to have small information sheets printed or photostated. This will save you from feeling like a gramophone. You might consider stating the following:

Protect all medicines from daylight.

Store in a cool, dark place, away from perfumes, mothballs and other aromatic substances.

Dissolve all medicines for oral use either on or under the tongue.

Crush all pills or tablets to a powder for small children.

Keep all medicines out of the reach of children (more as a matter of principle).

Do not eat or drink within fifteen minutes of taking an oral remedy.

Do not drink coffee, even the decaffeinated variety, whilst undergoing homoeopathic therapy. Substitute coffees, e.g. dandelion, are permissible.

Do not handle the remedies unnecessarily, e.g. to count them. Do not transfer them to another container.

Good luck!

5.

The Similimum

Both acute and chronic disease entities are treatable by the homoeopathic method. However, since the treatment of the chronic diseases is a rather more complex matter, we shall concentrate our initial discussions on the area of acute disease. It is in this field that you should gain your experience in prescribing. You then will be ready to tackle the chronic diseases. For the moment, you must have some patience.

Acute disease, by definition, tends to resolve spontaneously. Treatment is, however, desirable:

1. To reduce the discomfort of the patient
2. To encourage a rapid return to work or school.
3. To prevent the development of sequelae.

Even viral infections may be treated through homoeopathy. Whereas we have no antiviral, antibacterial, or antiparasitic agents as such, we do have remedies that stimulate the bodily response to such infections or infestations. The allopath works on the organism, the homoeopath on the host. Remedies have the ability to encourage the activity of the immune system. They must, however, be selected on the basis of the Law of Similars. That is to say, they must be *homoeopathic* to the disease. A remedy is *homoeopathic* to a disease when it has the potential to cause a *similar* disease in healthy subjects.

Hopefully, your initial exercise in prescribing is yielding results. You will recall that I termed this *simple* prescribing. By this I mean prescribing based on the correspondence (homoeopathicity) between a particular remedy and a particular orthodox diagnostic category. This is homoeopathic prescribing at its most basic level. In fact, the prescription of remedies must be based on the *individual* disease response.

Let me give you an example. Two children both have streptococcal tonsillitis. Their symptoms and signs, however, differ. They are *individualized:*

Child 1: High fever, delirium, red face, inflamed tonsils.

Child 2: Moderate fever, no delirium, severe otalgia, quinsy threatening.

In the first instance, the remedy is *Belladonna* (Deadly night-shade); in the second, *Mercurius solubilis* (Dimercurous ammonium nitrate).

Only where the human disease response tends to lack individualization — that is to say, where it is stereotyped — will there be a correspondence between one particular remedy and one allopathic disease entity. Such stereotyping of response does occur in those clinical situations given in your first exercise. This is the justification for the simple prescribing specified. This is why you should get reasonable results. However, in many other diagnostic categories, this simple approach would produce many failures. The human response is too variable. The remedy must be selected on the basis of individualized disease response.

Having said this, I do not want you to feel disheartened. There are ways around the problem. With respect to acute diseases, you should use the conventional diagnostic category, with which you are very familiar, as your starting point in remedy selection. For each allopathic category of disease, there will be, in general, a *small* number of common subtypes. Each subtype is determined by a certain complex of symptoms and signs. For each subtype, there will be a particular remedy homoeopathic to the complex. This is the so-called *similimum*. Under most circumstances, the presentation of disease in a particular patient can be readily matched with a common subtype, and the remedy deduced.

Let us take the four basic subtypes of *breast abscess* by way of example:

Type 1: Very early, pain and hardness just appearing. Pre-scription: Pilules *Bryonia* 6c (Wild hops), i each hour.

Type 2: Hardness less apparent, but red streaks radiate from a central point over the abscess. Prescription: Pilules *Belladonna* 6c, i each hour.

Type 3: Abscess has been developing for many hours, but frank pus formation (fluctuation) is not apparent. Prescription: Pilules *Phytolacca* 30c (Poke-root), i 4 hourly.

Type 4: Frank suppuration. Prescription: Pilules *Hepar sulphuris* 6c (an impure Calcium sulphide), i 4 hourly. Drainage may be required.

I have quoted the average potencies, and dose repetition for the sake of completeness, but, for the moment, disregard these matters. I would like you to appreciate that you must observe your patients carefully in order to be able to subtype them, and hence deduce the correct remedy, the *similimum*.

6.

Basic Remedies

Homoeopathy is very much concerned with the treatment of the patient as a whole. This will become more apparent when we pass to the treatment of the chronic diseases. The individualized disease response in the acute situation is determined in part by the general physio-anatomical make-up of the individual. The acute disease cannot be truly separated from the person in which it occurs. A knowledge of the person prior to the development of the acute disease may assist us in correct remedy selection, for it may well indicate a selection of remedies to which the patient is sensitive; that is to say, to which remedies he or she will most likely respond. For example, a young lady, of delicate emotional nature, with facial acne, late periods, and chronic catarrh, will be sensitive to the remedies *Pulsatilla* (Wind flower), and *Sulphur*. If she were to develop measles, one common subtype of which corresponds to *Pulsatilla*, then *Pulsatilla* would most likely be of great service in her acute therapy.

However, and fortunately for the beginner, excellent results can still be achieved *even if the constitutional base of the acute disease is ignored*. The matter of general make-up, or *constitution,* as it is termed, will be considered in our discussions on chronic disease.

For most situations, you will make effective prescriptions by noting the characteristics of the acute deviation from the norm of the patient.

Clarke's 'Prescriber'

Whereas it is my intention to provide you with sufficient prescribing information with respect to some common acute diseases, it will be necessary to acquire a satisfactory work of reference. *The Prescriber* by Dr John H. Clarke (Health Science Press) is strongly to be recommended. It will be found particularly of use for acute remedy selection, although it does have some excellent, though not entirely adequate, prescriptions for chronic disease. It conforms to the method of remedy selection that I have already suggested, viz. taking the conventional diagnosis as the starting point, and then determining the subtype.

The main problem for the beginner with *The Prescriber* is that the number of subtypes – and, therefore, suggested remedies – for many categories of disease seems a little excessive. Under 'Cough' alone, there are over forty subtypes! This is part of Clarke's natural thoroughness. This, of course, is tremendously useful for the professional homoeopathic physician, in prescribing with great accuracy, but is a little off-putting for the novice, not to mention extremely time-consuming. Besides, you may come up with a relatively rare remedy which neither you nor the local pharmacist has in stock.

As you will have anticipated, there are ways around this difficulty. The first thing to realize is that there is an overlap between the range of action of remedies. The second, that most homoeopathic basic work is carried out with a limited range of well-tried remedies. Whereas you may not have in stock the most homoeopathic remedy to the case, the *similimum*, you may be able to find a subtype of lesser similarity, which more-or-less corresponds to the case at hand, and for which the remedy is quickly available. For all practical purposes, the common remedy will act as the *similimum* for the case. Admittedly, it may not be as effective a therapeutic agent as the true *similimum*, but, nevertheless, much good work is done with such a compromise.

Therefore, when using *The Prescriber*, scan the subtypes for those that correspond to the major remedies. In most instances, you will find an acceptable similarity between one of these and the case at hand. Only proceed to the scrutiny of subtypes corresponding to obscure remedies if desperate.

You must, therefore, be familiar with the major and commonly used remedies in acute homoeopathy. You must arrange to stock them yourself, or for the local pharmacist to stock them on your behalf. They are:

Acidum phosphoricum (Phosphoric acid)
Aconite (Monkshood)
Antimonium tartaricum (Tartar emetic)
Apis mellifica (The honey-bee)
Arnica montana
Arsenicum album (Arsenic trioxide)
Bach Rescue Remedy
Baptisia (Wild indigo)
Belladonna

Bryonia
Calcarea carbonica (Carbonate of lime)
Calendula
Cantharis (Spanish fly)
Carbo vegetabilis (Vegetable charcoal)
Colocynthis (Bitter cucumber)
Drosera (Sundew)
Ferrum phosphoricum (Phosphate of Iron)
Gelsemium (Yellow jasmine)
Gunpowder
Hepar sulph.
Hypericum (St John's wort)
Ipecacuanha (Ipecac-root)
Kali. bichromicum (Potassium bichromate)
Mercurius sol.
Natrum muriaticum (Rock-salt)
Nux vomica
Oscillococcinum (prepared from infected duck tissue)
Phytolacca
Pulsatilla
Pyrogen (Artificial sepsin)
Phosphorus
Silicea
Spongia tosta (Roasted common sponge)
Sulphur

Thirty four remedies in all. These will provide enough therapeutic range for the bulk of early prescribing in acute disease. *Bach Rescue Remedy* is stocked as drops, *Calendula* as 5% cream, the remainder as pilules or tablets. The most convenient potencies are either 6c or 30c, but *Gunpowder* should be stocked in 6x potency (as compressed tablets of the trituration), *Oscillococcinum* in 200c, and *Bach Rescue Remedy* is essentially a Ø. Obviously, other remedies, such as *Euphrasia,* will be required from time to time, and these are mentioned throughout the text. These may be added at leisure to the basic stock.

You will also find within *The Prescriber* useful suggestions as to potency and dose repetition. Clarke, however, used a wide range of potencies. You will find, nevertheless, that the bulk of your work can be successfully accomplished with either 6c or 30c. Where Clarke suggests potencies in the range 1c to 6c, use 6c. For the range 12c to 200c, use 30c. In your first exercise, you will recall that I suggested that the potency of *Euphrasia* should be 12c. Let us suppose that you only have the 30c. Since 30c is a little *more* potent than 12c, it is prescribed a little less frequently, say bd instead of tid. If you only have the 6c, which is a little *less* potent than the 30c, prescribe it more frequently, say qid.

For correct remedy selection, you will require the following details with regard to the acute deviation:

1. The conventional diagnosis. This defines the pathology and its site. Only where the human response is stereotyped (e.g. traumatic bruising) will this provide us with enough information to select the similimum. It does, however, provide us with a limited number of therapeutic possibilities.

2. The actual signs and symptoms as manifest in the particular patient. If there is swelling, whether hard or soft, whether pale or erythematous. If there is pain, its site, its radiation, and its quality (pricking, dull, aching, burning, electric, etc.). Is there a fever, and to what degree? Is the patient thirsty or thirstless? Is the patient flushed, or sweaty? And so on. These points are most important in determining the *individualization* of disease, and, therefore, enable us to match the case to an appropriate subtype, and hence find the appropriate similimum. Symptoms may be either *local* or *concomitant*. *Local symptoms* are those related to the site of the pathology. *Concomitant symptoms* are those which occur distantly from the site of the pathology, though are connected with the acute illness. Hence, a throbbing frontal headache accompanying acute tonsillitis may be regarded as a concomitant symptom. Such concomitant symptoms are of great use in selecting the appropriate subtype.

3. The *modalities*. These are those things that make the patient either better or worse. They include: temperature variation, stuffy atmospheres, weather, drinking, eating, micturition, and so on. In homoeopathic textbooks, the sign < means 'worse for/from', and the sign >, 'better for/from'. Hence, '< stuffy atmosphere' means '*worse* from stuffy atmosphere'; and '> lying down' means '*better* for lying down'. Also to be included in this category are the time modalities; that is to say, at what particular times the patient feels better or worse. The assessment of modalities is of great importance in the selection of remedies. For example, the modalities:

worse from wet weather, after midnight, from cold or cold drinks.

better from heat, head elevated, warm drinks tend to suggest the remedy *Arsenicum album*.

4. The *causation*. By this we mean the circumstances that brought on the illness. This often expedites remedy selection, for certain remedies have a pronounced correspondence to certain types of causation. For example, *Aconite* for ailments brought on by sudden chilling (cold winds or draughts), and *Ignatia* (St Ignatius bean) for ailments brought on by fright, or grief.

Together, these facts constitute what is termed the *totality* of the acute disease.

During epidemics of acute infectious disease it is often observable that the majority of cases show considerable similarity in their totality. This totality, peculiar to the particular epidemic, is termed the *genus epidemicus*. In correspondence, a particular remedy will be found that bears a homoeopathic relationship to the *genus*. Thus, in a recent viral epidemic, the majority of patients experienced the irritating accumulation of mucus in the posterior nares, with much coughing, followed by retching or vomiting. In this instance the *genus epidemicus* corresponded to the remedy *Ipecacuanha*. Determination of the *genus,* and hence the appropriate remedy during epidemic outbreaks serves to simplify prescribing. In this way large numbers of cases can be simply and swiftly treated. Furthermore, the same remedy may be used in a preventative manner in order to limit spread of the disease throughout the population. It must be realized, however, that cases which lack similarity to the *genus* must be treated with other remedies.

7.
Home Remedy Kits

You now realize, with respect to the conventional diagnostic category, that the human response may be stereotypic or diverse. Your next clinical exercise involves the prescription of *home remedy kits*. These contain a selected number of remedies for the use of patients at home for the treatment of some common acute complaints. They depend for their efficacy on the following fundamental facts:

1. That the human response is stereotyped with regard to certain conventional diagnoses.

2. That, where the human response is diverse, a particular subtype is the most common, and, therefore, a particular remedy is most commonly indicated.

Home remedy kits should be issued to your more interested patients with young families. Your local health visitor will probably assist you in their selection. The home remedy kit may be as long, or as short, as a piece of string, but the following one, containing eleven remedies, will be found to be fairly useful:

ABC 30c (*Aconite* 30 + *Belladonna* 30 + *Chamomilla* 30), 7g pilules.

Oscillococcinum 200c (prepared from duck's liver), 7g pilules.

Urtica urens 6c, 7g pilules.

Gunpowder 6x, 7g tablets.

Arsenicum album 6c, 7g pilules.

Nux vomica 6c, 7g pilules.

Arnica montana 30c, 7g pilules.

Antimonium tart. 6c, 7g pilules.

Apis mel. 6c, 7g pilules.

Calendula ∅ 5% cream, 35g.

Bach Rescue Remedy, 5ml in dropper bottle.

Each home remedy kit should be supplied complete with a basic instruction sheet. It is a useful exercise to compose the latter personally. It should contain the general information with regard to administration and protection of remedies, and also give the principal indications for each remedy, and the average frequency of dose repetition. *Arnica* and *Calendula* have been discussed previously.

ABC 30, as indicated, is a mixture of three remedies which have been separately potentized. It is *not* produced by mixing three Ø, and subsequently potentizing them together. This is an extremely good, and well-tried, mixture for fevers and teething problems. The patient may be given one pilule every half hour until the temperature begins to fall, or the inquietude and fractious disturbance of teething settles. This is the key remedy for the fever state in childhood.

It is not, however, as it might seem on the surface, a mere symptomatic treatment. It does not merely reduce the fever. It treats the underlying disease that gives rise to the fever. It promotes the bodily reaction against what is usually an infecting organism, and thus causes the fever to fall. Conventional treatment with acetylsalicylic acid may prevent the occurrence of febrile convulsion, but it must be remembered that the febrile state itself is to some degree protective, in that it is inhibitory to micro-organisms. Acetylsalicylic acid does not enhance the bodily reactivity, whilst *ABC* does.

The matter of *polypharmacy* requires some discussion. After all, one of the great criticisms of allopathic practice has been the use of multiple drugs simultaneously, and the generation thereby of problematical side-effects. Similarly, there are many physicians who frown upon homoeopathic polypharmacy, since they declare that only a single remedy (the *similimum*) should be given at one time, for an inimical or antidotal relationship may exist between simultaneously administered remedies. However, it is an established clinical fact that certain mixtures of remedies, such as *ABC* 30, are highly effective therapeutically, and neither produce an inimical nor antidotal effect. In the face of this clinical evidence, and bearing in mind that the object of homoeopathic polypharmacy is to broaden the therapeutic range of a medicine so that it is more simply prescribed, there should be little objection to the use of well-tried mixtures. Any such objections are based upon ignorance of the practical facts.

Let us take a brief look at the three components of *ABC*. *Aconite* treats ailments of sudden onset brought on by chilling. It is, therefore, of great use at the commencement of common colds. In its *provings,* that is to say its effects on healthy subjects, it produces great *fear*. It is not surprising, therefore, that it is of great service in those states that cause great fear, such as road traffic accident, or myocardial infarction. Even if *Aconite* is not available on its own, *ABC* may be given in such fearful states with equal effect. *Belladonna* in its provings produces a state that most closely resembles scarlet fever, and is thus homoeopathic to many cases of this disease. It will, however, be found of service in most febrile states characterized by flushing of the face, throbbing headache and delirium. Similarly, it helps the sufferer from sunstroke. *Chamomilla* is probably the most useful remedy in teething problems: fractious behaviour, child wishes to be carried, diarrhoea from teething, teething fevers.

Thus, *ABC* may be of service in many febrile illnesses, states causing great fear, teething problems, or sunstroke. Occasionally, it will actually abort an infective problem, if given early enough in the course of a disease. More usually, with regard to fevers, the temperature will fall, and another remedy must be introduced subsequently to assist the healing process. If the fever should rise again, do not be afraid to repeat *ABC*. However, there will be some rare instances where it fails to control the temperature, and both you and the parents begin to panic as the child's temperature shoots past 103°F. Here, you should suggest tepid spongeing, whilst you select a remedy more homoeopathic to the case, such as *Mercurius sol.* for acute otitis media. These matters will be discussed later. In the case of great sepsis, such as severe acute tonsillitis, where *ABC* is inadequate, *Pyrogen* 30 (a nosode) given half-hourly will often rescue the situation.

Oscillococcinum is a *nosode*. The term *nosode* applies to any remedy prepared from micro-organisms, or infected tissue, and is thus akin to the notion of a *vaccine* in allopathic medicine. *Oscillococcinum* is prepared from infected duck tissue. It heightens the immune response to many common viral infections, including the common cold, and influenza. It may be given routinely, therefore, in such ailments in a dosage of one pilule every four hours. In my experience, it has no adverse interreaction with other remedies given commonly in the treatment of such states. In fact, I generally administer it along with the classically indicated homoeopathic remedy. Even in the absence of complementary (synergistic) remedies, *Oscillococcinum* may do yeoman work. In some cases, it may be used preventatively, moreover. To prevent recurrent viral infections, or to reduce their intensity, should they occur. In these instances, it may be prescribed in a dosage of one pilule twice weekly (e.g. Monday and Thursday evenings). We shall have more to say of the treatment of *predisposition* in our deliberations over chronic disease, for the predisposition to recurrent infection is truly a manifestation of an underlying chronic disease.

Urtica is of assistance when given internally for burns. The initial dosage should be one pilule every fifteen minutes, reducing to one every hour or two, as the symptoms wane. Externally, *Calendula* cream from the kit should be applied. In the absence of *Calendula,* the oily contents of a Vitamin E capsule may be applied to the burn. Vitamin E used in this fashion rapidly promotes healing.

Gunpowder is of great service in the treatment of furuncles. The dosage is one tablet 4-hourly. If, however, we are able to catch the boil at its very early stage of development, when it is red, swollen, throbbing, and frank pus has not yet formed, then *Belladonna* is well indicated. *Belladonna* is given 2-hourly. *ABC* may be used alternatively, since it contains this remedy.

Arsenicum album, one pilule 4-hourly, may be used for gastroenteritis.

Nux vomica, one pilule 4-hourly, assists in largely gastric upsets, such as 'the morning after the night before' syndrome.

Antimonium tart., one pilule thrice daily is of great service in many cases of acute bronchitis, where there is much rattling of mucus.

Apis mel., given in a dosage of one pilule every ten minutes initially, is used to treat insect stings.

Rescue Remedy belongs to a group of extremely valuable remedies devised by Dr E. Bach, and known as the *Bach Flower Remedies*. They are essentially macerations of plant material in brandy, the insoluble material having been filtered out, and do not carry a potency symbol. As a group they are of great therapeutic value in the treatment of mental and psychosomatic illness, and will require further close scrutiny in this respect. *Rescue Remedy* itself is a mixture of five of the Flower Remedies: *Star of Bethlehem,* for shock; *Rock Rose,* for terror and panic; *Impatiens,* for mental stress and tension; *Cherry Plum,* for desperation; and *Clematis* for the depersonalization that occurs prior to loss of consciousness. *Rescue Remedy* has probably saved many lives. It may be used in any situation where there is sudden mental or physical shock, e.g. the ill-effects of an accident, hearing bad news, sudden onset of asthma, myocardial infarction. It is given in drop form, two or three drops constituting a single dose, and these may be given in a tablespoon of water, or directly on to the tongue of the patient. In severe conditions, such as myocardial infarction, the dose may be repeated as often as every two minutes. In lesser conditions, repeat every ten minutes until the patient improves. With regard to asthma, it certainly seems to take the edge off the anxiety component, but is often insufficient in itself to completely abort the attack.

You will discover, I think, that the home remedy kit is an extremely useful adjunct to general practice. Make it your business to find out how your patients are getting on with their remedies. The sensible use of such methods reduces the frequency of visits to the doctor for many common ailments.

The home remedy kit is a simple and effective instrument by which both patient and physician can learn the properties of remedies, and their common application.

8.

Prescribing in Acute Disease

It must be emphasized that homoeopathic remedies do not merely remove symptoms. That the symptoms of the patient must guide us in our choice of remedy is obvious, yet the appropriate remedy exerts its influence on the disease process itself. In this way are the symptoms removed. Thus, homoeopathy is not guilty of what is termed the *suppression* of disease. It does not sweep the dust under the carpet!

Neither is it true that the homoeopathic physician is unconcerned with the results of modern investigative techniques. Pathological investigation is just as much a part of homoeopathy as it is of allopathy. It is the treatment that is different. The results of such investigations may guide us towards the selection of the *similimum*. A positive blood test for glandular fever, for example, will place the remedy *Glandular Fever Nosode* high on the list of possible therapeutic agents. The presence in the blood of granulocytosis in the course of a severe infective illness will make us think of *Pyrogen,* and so on.

Thus, homoeopathy moves with the times. It may appear to some as a revivalist art of archaic structure, yet nothing could be further from the truth. It is a dynamic and progressive system of modern medicine.

Now, many physicians are put off homoeopathy because it would seem that the selection of the *similimum* is a most complex task. The implication of many texts is that a 'bull's eye' must be scored every time for victory. However, it is a clinical fact that most therapeutic victories in the treatment of patients suffering from acute diseases are won with non-perfect scores. That is to say, much good work is done with partially-matched remedies, and this particularly so in the case of children, with their highly responsive immune systems. Moreover, as I was once taught by a most distinguished allopathic specialist, *common things occur commonly.* Commonly used remedies are commonly effective in common diseases.

In the dialogues that follow, we shall be discussing the treatment of a variety of common acute disease situations, before we pass to the treatment of chronic disease. You will observe not only that there may be several remedies for each conventional diagnostic category (each one corresponding to a particular subtype), but that certain remedies are of service in the treatment of several different categories of disease. These remedies of wide clinical application are termed *polychrests*. They include such great remedies as *Phosphorus* and *Sulphur*.

Throughout, I have taken the liberty of suggesting potency and average dose repetition. These matters are, however, not inflexible, and may be modified in each individual case. This, however, is a matter of experience, and, for the moment, it would be better to follow these guidelines. Concerning the matter of dose repetition, it will become apparent that this is largely determined by the severity of the disease at hand. It may vary from once every two minutes, in the case of the collapsed patient, to twice daily, in the case of a lingering viral infection. In all cases, as improvement sets in, one must be prepared to reduce the frequency of the dosage. In cases where the disease evolves into a new symptomatic picture, the practitioner must be prepared to change course, and prescribe a different remedy in correspondence to the new clinical entity.

Having found your feet through the clinical exercises given previously, and through the application of the home remedy kit, it is now your responsibility to plunge deeper into the subject of homoeopathy. This may be achieved by following the therapeutic principles outlined.

In order to avoid repetition, I shall assume that you now realize that a single dose corresponds to one pilule, one tablet, or 1-3 drops of liquid potency or Ø.

9.

Fever and Acute Otitis Media

A child presents with a FEVER. As yet, there are no localizing signs. Do we wait, or do we treat? We treat, for by so doing we may halt the disease abruptly, or at least reduce its severity. Think first of *Aconite* 30, ½-hourly, until the temperature falls. Alternatively, *ABC* 30, ½-hourly. As I have said previously, *Aconite* is particularly useful in ailments brought on by sudden chilling, an event which lowers the bodily resistance to infection. Concurrently, you may give *Oscillococcinum* 200, 4-hourly, if a viral infection is suspected.

A child presents with FEVER PLUS OTALGIA. Initially, use *Aconite* or *ABC* again. But a frank ACUTE OTITIS MEDIA develops. Switch to *Mercurius sol.* 30, 2-hourly, reducing the dose interval to 4-hourly or 6-hourly as improvement occurs. *Mercurius sol.* is almost specific for acute otitis media, and often works faster than any antibiotic. Even if ACUTE TONSILLITIS is present concurrently with the ear infection, still think of *Mercurius sol.*

Another remedy of great use in early ear infections, and indeed in early inflammations anywhere, prior to the stage of frank exudation, is *Ferrum phos.* Give *Ferrum phos.* 30, 2-hourly. This remedy, given ½-hourly, will also deal with a large proportion of ACUTE EPISTAXES. The homoeopathic treatment of ear infections may be complemented by the use of *garlic,* a substance with peculiar antibiotic properties. It may be given in the form of tablets or capsules, i bd. For very small children, or those who are reluctant to take oral garlic, a crushed clove of the latter may be placed in a sock and applied to the skin of the foot. From this site, there is rapid transcutaneous absorption. This method may, indeed, be used in the presence of any infection of the upper or lower respiratory tract, often to great effect.

Effective prescribing prevents rupture of the tympanic membrane. But, let us suppose a child arrives in the surgery with pus pouring fourth from the middle ear. What then? Prescribe *Calcarea carb.* 6, thrice daily, or, alternatively, *Hepar sulph.* 6, thrice daily, until the ear is dry.

Finally, after the acute infection subsides, we are left with a lingering eustachian catarrh, with some deafness, and popping noises in the ear. *Kali. mur.* 6, thrice daily, administered from several days to two weeks, will usually clear this problem. Also, never forget the value of steam in loosening tenacious mucus.

10.

Colds, Influenza
and Respiratory Infection

The COMMON COLD is best treated at its very onset, in order to stop it dead in its tracks. Use *Aconite* 30, 2-hourly, if brought on by chilling, and *Oscillococcinum* 200, 4-hourly, in all cases. Where a cold commences with sneezing, use *Natrum mur.* 30, 2-hourly. Additionally, extra vitamin C, several grams daily, and garlic may be helpful.

However, once a cold has been allowed to develop, it becomes a veritable symptomatic chameleon. Using classical homoeopathic methods to treat this illness is both complex and tedious. Within a few hours of prescribing a classical remedy (e.g. *Nux vomica* 30, 2-hourly, for a stuffed-up nose), the disease has a nasty habit of changing its character, moving out of the sphere of action of the previous remedy, and requiring the application of a new remedy. Fortunately, in many cases, the problem is overcome by utilizing a single remedy, *Oscillococcinum* 200, 4-hourly, throughout the illness; and this may be combined effectively with vitamin C and garlic therapy as mentioned previously.

INFLUENZA, in its very earliest stages, may be arrested by the timely administration of *Influenzinum Co.* 30, 4-hourly. Once it has developed, it tends not to have the same chameleon-like behaviour of the common cold, and, thus, classical remedies are more simply applied. Where there is general prostration, muscular weakness, and severe occipital headache, *Gelsemium* 30, 2-hourly, should be given. Where there is generalized muscular soreness, *Baptisia* 30, 2-hourly, is better indicated. Where there is great aching of the bones, as well as the flesh, prescribe *Eupatorium perfoliatum* 30 (Thoroughwort), 2-hourly. Throughout, complementary treatment with vitamin C, garlic, and either *Oscillococcinum* 200 or *Influenzinum Co.* 30, 4-hourly, is helpful.

As a complication of a cold or influenza, ACUTE BRONCHITIS develops. At the very earliest stage, a few doses of *Ferrum phos.* 30, or *Phosphorus* 30, 4-hourly, may abort the descent of the infection. The dry cough of early tracheitis or bronchitis — especially if the patient is thirsty, the chest is sore, and the cough is worse for entering a warm room — is usually treated with *Bryonia* 30, 4-hourly; and this may be used in 2-hourly alternation with *Phosphorus* (e.g. 8 a.m.: *Phosphorus;* 10 a.m.: *Bryonia;* 12 midday: *Phosphorus,* etc.). Where the chest develops frank râles ('rattly chest'), then *Antimonium tart.* 30, 4-hourly, is often indicated. Where nausea accompanies the cough, *Ipecacuanha* 30, 4-hourly, is of service in many cases.

Where INFANTILE CROUP develops, steam should be applied immediately. Additionally, the following three remedies should be applied in the order specified, in alternation, every ten minutes: *Aconite* 30, *Hepar sulph.* 30, *Spongia tosta* 30.

General debility following influenza usually responds to either *Gelsemium* 30, or *Acidum phos.* 30, bd. Persistent green catarrh following viral infections may be treated with either *Kali. bich.* 30, or *Pulsatilla* 30, bd.

11.

The Ill-effects of Antibiotics

Antibiotics are the most misused and overused drugs of modern allopathic practice. The ILL-EFFECTS OF ANTIBIOTICS stem largely from their interference with the balance of the normal alimentary flora. The patient may develop malaise, gastro-intestinal disturbance, or thrush. In all such cases it is advisable to prescribe one small carton of yogurt daily (goat's yogurt for those allergic to cow's milk), and garlic tablets or capsules, ii bd for adults, and i bd for children. Infants may be given generous quantities of garlic in their diet. The combination of garlic and yogurt assists in the restoration of the floral imbalance.

Additionally, where diarrhoea stems from the administration of antibiotics, prescribe *Acidum nit*. 30 (Nitric acid), bd. Where oral or vaginal THRUSH develops, prescribe *Borax* 30, tid. *Borax* is a good all-round remedy for thrush, whatever the cause.

Where a cutaneous allergic response arises as the result of the administration of antibiotics, or, for that matter, any drug, then it is wise, after stopping the drug, to give *Sulphur* 6, once daily. Placing the patient with DRUG RASH on a total fruit juice elimination diet for several days assists in the removal of the offending drug, and the toxic products of the allergic response.

12.

Specific Infectious
Fevers of Childhood

The SPECIFIC INFECTIOUS FEVERS OF CHILDHOOD are readily treated with remedies, in order to improve the comfort of the patient, shorten the duration of the illness, and prevent the development of serious sequelae. In all, at their very commencement, *Aconite* 30, $\frac{1}{2}$-2-hourly, may be given, until the symptomatic picture clarifies. Also, *Oscillococcinum* 200, 4-hourly, if there is a good chance that we might be dealing with a common cold or influenza. If the overt disease then develops, we must resort to other remedial measures.

For WHOOPING COUGH, *Pertussin* 30, bd. Additionally, *Drosera* 30, 4-hourly, especially if the cough is worse after midnight. Prescribe *Ipecacuanha* 30, 4-hourly, if there is much vomiting.

For SCARLET FEVER, *Belladonna* 30, 4-hourly, is almost specific.

For MEASLES, *Morbillinum* 30, bd, and, in many cases, *Pulsatilla* 30, 4-hourly. *Euphrasia* 30, 4-hourly, may be required if conjunctivitis is a dominant feature.

GERMAN MEASLES is usually a mild illness requiring little medicinal treatment, except *ABC* 30, 4-hourly. The administration of remedies *enhances* the immune response. Long-lasting immunity to rubella is not, therefore, impaired by remedial application.

For MUMPS, *Parotidinum* 30, bd. Additionally, in general, *Jaborandi* 30 (Pilocarpus micro.), 4-hourly. Where orchitis occurs concomitantly, *Pulsatilla* 30, 4-hourly.

For CHICKEN-POX, in the vesicular stage, either *Antimonium tart.* 30, or *Rhus tox.* 30, 4-hourly. When general improvement sets in, *Mercurius sol.* 30, bd.

For GLANDULAR FEVER, *Glandular fever nosode* 30, bd, is often of great service.

For STREPTOCOCCAL TONSILLITIS, *Mercurius sol.* 30, 4-hourly, deals with many cases, even if a QUINSY is threatening. Where there is a marked lymphadenitis, use *Phytolacca* 30, 4-hourly.

For ACUTE HERPETIC GINGIVOSTOMATITIS, with foul breath and excessive salivation, prescribe *Mercurius sol*. 30, tid. If, however, the mouth is dry, and there is much prostration, then *Baptisia* 30, tid, is better indicated.

13.
Homoeopathic
Preventative Medicine

Homoeopathic remedies may be used to great effect in the prevention of acute infection. These measures are of particular importance during epidemics, or to prevent infection spreading from one member of a household to another. This is one aspect of HOMOEOPATHIC PREVENTATIVE MEDICINE. As with their conventional counterparts, homoeopathic immunization techniques may have their failures, but these seem to be rare. Moreover, should the patient develop the disease, the case would appear to be milder and more manageable than would be normally anticipated. The following remedies should all be given once weekly. Occasional reactions do occur with initial dosages, but these are mild (e.g. runny nose), and of little consequence. As with other remedies, the oral route is preferred.

Disease	Preventative remedy
Whooping-cough	*Pertussin* 30
Measles	*Morbillinum* 30
Mumps	*Parotidinum* 30
Influenza	*Influenzinum Co.* 30
Chicken-pox	*Varicella* 30
Common cold	*Oscillococcinum* 200

It would be a mistake, however, to merely rely upon specific immunization techniques, whether they be homoeopathic, utilizing the above nosodes derived from appropriate organisms, or allopathic. The general health of the patient is of equal importance in determining the degree of immunity conferred. The general resistance of the patient must be of the highest order. This involves the provision of a satisfactory diet, and the correction, with remedies, of any constitutional weaknesses. These matters will be discussed more fully with regard to the matter of chronic disease. Homoeopathy has a lot more to offer than mere specific protection.

The concept of prevention in homoeopathy is, however, wider than this. We may, for example, prevent SEA-SICKNESS in susceptible individuals by prescribing either *Cocculus indicus* 30 (Indian cockle), or *Petroleum* 30, 6-hourly for two days prior to the voyage, and every hour during the voyage. We may prevent examination failure in capable but nervous persons by prescribing appropriate remedies, and the same may be utilized to prevent the TREPIDATION that precedes hospitalization, or a visit to the dental surgeon. Where the patient would normally suffer, under such circumstances, from loss of memory, weakness of the legs, diarrhoea, drowsiness, give *Gelsemium* 30, bd for several days prior to the event, and an extra dose on the day. Where the patient would suffer from agitation, diarrhoea, hurried actions, incessant speech, give *Argentum nitricum* 30 (Silver nitrate), in like dosage. The largely hypokinetic picture of the *Gelsemium* patient contrasts sharply with the hyperkinetic picture of his *Argentum nitricum* counterpart.

14.
Sequential, Concurrent and Alternate Prescribing

You will have gathered that there are four different ways in which it is possible to prescribe different remedies in a particular case:

1. *Sequentially.* Only a single remedy is prescribed at one time. The change to the next single remedy (the second *similimum*) being determined by a definite change in the subjective and objective symptomatic picture.

2. *Concurrently.* Two or more remedies are prescribed together, sometimes in a preprepared combination, e.g. *ABC.*

3. *Concurrently and sequentially.* A basic remedy (e.g. *Oscillococcinum*) is prescribed throughout the treatment, but the concurrent remedies are changed as the subjective and objective symptomatic picture alters.

4. *Alternately.* Two or more remedies are prescribed in alternation, there being a definite interval (from ten minutes, to several hours) between the application of each remedy.

Another variant, involving sequential prescription, is to change potency. A case of acute tonsillitis may respond partially to *Mercurius sol.* 6, 4-hourly. We increase the dose repetition to 2-hourly, but little extra benefit is obtained. Because we feel that the symptomatic picture still justifies the use of the same remedy, it is advisable to prescribe a higher potency. Thus, we now prescribe *Mercurius sol.* 30, 4-hourly.

Sequential prescribing is both the classical method, and the simplest for the newcomer to homoeopathy. It does, however, suffer from the disadvantage of delay, where either an incorrect remedy or incorrect potency has been selected. This is obviously more likely to happen in early ventures into homoeopathic prescribing, but it is to be remembered that even experienced prescribers are not infallible. The matter of delay is of little consequence in many cases, but others are of sufficient gravity to warrant a more certain approach to therapy.

To these ends, the methods of concurrent and alternate prescribing have been introduced into modern homoeopathy. *Concurrent* prescribing, however, is not without problems. These stem from the fact that certain remedies have either an *antidotal* or *inimical* relationship. That is to say, they either antidote each other's therapeutic action completely or partially, or they are totally incompatible, with the production of some undesirable, though seldom particularly harmful, reaction. Thus *Mercurius sol.* and *Silicea* should not be used together, since they are inimical. *Alternate* prescribing largely avoids any such complications.

You may take it, that where specified as acceptable and efficaceous in reputable works of reference, the method of concurrent prescription may be used. If, however, after taking the case, you are split between two different remedies, and you can find no reference to the acceptability of their concurrent usage, then it is best to prescribe them in alternation. If, to take the matter one stage further, the case is of such urgency, that you feel it would be best to prescribe the different remedies simultaneously, then you must consult a work of reference that delineates the relationship of remedies. The easiest to use is the *Relationship of Remedies* by Dr R. Gibson Miller. With great rapidity, you will be able to determine whether the remedies in question have either an antidotal or inimical relationship. If they do, you must think again. If such a relationship is not recorded, then, in most cases, you may assume that their concurrent prescription is unlikely to cause any problems. This at least is true with the prescription concurrently of two remedies, but with three or more remedies, it may not be so. This is why, except in very special instances, such as the use of *ABC,* you are not at liberty, in general, to administer complex multiple mixtures to cover all possible eventualities. Even if not inimical in relationship, the contents of such complex mixtures frequently are antidotal. They should not be used, unless it has been demonstrated that they are effective.

Before we pass back to particular therapies, one small fact is worthy of note. Just occasionally, the administration of a remedy is followed by a slight apparent worsening of the patient's condition. This is termed a *healing crisis,* and more shall be said of this with regard to chronic disease treatment. Unlike a real worsening of the patient's condition, it is short-lived, and followed by an improvement (healing) phase. Thus, the sore throat of acute tonsillitis may worsen for say thirty minutes after taking *Mercurius sol.,* only to be followed by a rapid recovery phase. The precaution you must take, so as not to overstimulate the healing response, is to withhold the remedy as long as the patient continues to improve. The remedy should only be reapplied if the improvement plateaus out short of cure. In those cases where a healing crisis is not well-tolerated by the patient, the prescription of the remedy subsequently is advised in a lesser potency. Hence, where a potency of 30 has caused a healing crisis, a 6 may be prescribed subsequently.

15.

Sudden Collapse

It is often erroneously thought that homoeopathy is only suited to the treatment of minor complaints. Nothing could be further from the truth. Indeed, the correct application of remedies in serious situations has been known to save lives. SUDDEN COLLAPSE from whatever cause, be it a simple vasovagal attack or myocardial infarction, should, in addition to the usual resuscitative measures, receive the benefit of remedial prescription.

Bach Rescue Remedy is a complex mixture of proven clinical efficacy. *It should be carried by every physician in his emergency bag.* It is not adequate merely to have the chemist stock it on your behalf. In *all* cases of sudden collapse, three drops, every two minutes, should be administered directly on to the tongue of the patient until recovery occurs. Additionally, *Carbo veg.* 30, a single dose as soon as possible. This may be administered as drops, or a single pulverised pilule or tablet. *Carbo veg.* has been called, perhaps with a little exaggeration, 'the homoeopathic corpse reviver'.

In cases of acute myocardial infarction, where the patient is not collapsed, but complains of severe chest pain, the same remedial methods should be applied. However, either *Latrodectus mactans* 30 (Black widow spider), or *Cactus grandiflorus* 30 (Night-blooming Cereus) should be administered every ten minutes in addition to the former measures. These may be of some assistance in the control of pain. These two remedies are also of use in the control of ANGINA PECTORIS. Here the dosage would be one pilule or tablet every two minutes until the pain is relieved.

In cases of sudden collapse associated with loss of vital fluids (gastro-intestinal fluids, serum, blood), *China* 30, $\frac{1}{4}$-hourly, is indicated.

16.

Infective Disease of the Skin

BOILS may be treated in their early stages, when there is little swelling, but redness and much throbbing, with *Belladonna* 30, 2-hourly. Alternatively, *Gunpowder* 6x, 4-hourly. Once frank pus has formed, as witnessed by fluctuation or the appearance of a pustular head, then it is more fitting to prescribe *Hepar sulph.* 6, 4-hourly, in order to promote discharge. In those instances where incision would seem indicated, but, as in the case of a child, one would prefer to avoid the scalpel, then give *Myristica* 3x (Brazilian ucuba), hourly. Once pus has discharged, use *Silicea* 6, bd, to encourage rapid healing. DENTAL ABSCESS may be treated along similar lines, but also requires the advice of a dental surgeon.

CARBUNCLES often respond to *Tarentula cubensis* 30 (Cuban spider), tid. Where BOILS are RECURRENT. a few doses of *Anthracinum* 200 (Anthrax nosode), bd, will usually arrest them.

CELLULITIS, in its early stages, may be treated with *Apis mell.* 30, 2-hourly. When red and throbbing, with *Belladonna* 30, 4-hourly. When bluish in colour, *Lachesis* 30 (Bushmaster venom), 4-hourly.

IMPETIGO is treated with *Antimonium crudum* 6 (Black sulphide of Antimony), 4-hourly. This deals with most cases, and, furthermore, is of great service in the treatment of superimposed infection upon eczema.

For INGROWING TOENAIL infection, *Magnetis pol. aust.* 30 (South pole of magnet), bd, is virtually specific.

HERPES LABIALIS generally responds to either *Natrum mur.* 30, or *Rhus tox.* 30 (Poison ivy), tid. Recurrent cases will require chronic disease therapy as discussed later. HERPES ZOSTER may also require the action of *Rhus tox.* 30, tid.

17.

Acute Orthopaedic Problems

Acute ORTHOPAEDIC problems are commonly seen in general practice. Homoeopathic remedies will be found extremely useful as therapeutic adjuvants. The use of *Arnica* for acute sprains has already been mentioned, and no remedy is its superior with respect to such injuries.

For PULLED MUSCLES, use a 2-hourly alternation of *Arnica* 30 and *Rhus tox.* 30. For simple extreme muscular fatigue following vigorous exercise, *Arnica* 30, hourly.

TENNIS ELBOW usually responds to *Ruta* 6, tid. The same remedy, in similar potency, may be used to treat SPRAINED WRIST, after *Arnica* has been used for a day or two, ACUTE EYE-STRAIN with accompanying headache, and CONTUSIONS OF BONES. *Ruta* 6, bd, is also of use in the treatment of NON-UNION of fractures. Were *Symphytum* 6x (Comfrey), bd, given routinely for *all* fracture cases, for it promotes union with great efficacy, then non-union might occur less frequently. What cheaper medicines could there be than Rue (*Ruta*) and Comfrey?

Acute WRY-NECK, from sitting in a draught may respond to *Aconite* 30, hourly. STIFF BACKS that loosen with mobility often respond to *Rhus tox.* 30, tid. ACUTE SCIATICA usually requires the intervention of osteopathy or acupuncture for swift relief, the application of remedies being valuable, but of secondary importance.

18.

Acute Abdominal Complaints

ACUTE GASTRO-ENTERITIS, including that which stems from food poisoning, frequently responds to *Arsenicum album* 30, tid. Simple gastric irritation from change in diet, or dietary indiscretion, should usually succumb to *Nux vomica* 30, hourly.

Severe abdominal COLIC, from whatever cause, prior to the establishment of a surgical diagnosis, when the characteristic modality 'better for doubling up' is present, should be treated with either *Colocynthis* 30, or *Magnesia phos*. 30 (Magnesium phosphate), $\frac{1}{4}$-hourly. These remedies induce relaxation of smooth muscle, and thus treat the underlying cause of the pain. They are not, therefore, to be regarded as agents which mask the disease, but as agents of therapy. *Mag. phos*. is also of service in the treatment of menstrual colic.

Generalized abdominal distention, discomfort, and flatulence, accompanying SUBACUTE BOWEL OBSTRUCTION due to adhesions may be treated with *China* 30 (Peruvian bark), 2-hourly.

The majority of cases of ACUTE CYSTITIS in women respond to *Cantharis* 30, tid.

19.

Pregnancy and Lactation

The use of allopathic medicines in PREGNANCY, for fear of harm befalling the foetus, is generally and wisely proscribed. In contrast, because of their lack of toxicity, homoeopathic remedies may be freely prescribed with impunity, both for matters directly concerned with gestation and parturition, and diseases occurring during pregnancy, though not directly related to it. The only modification to be made to this statement is with regard to the matter of homoeopathic aggravation, or healing crisis, as it is termed. Though of infrequent occurrence with respect to the treatment of acute disease, it does, nevertheless, occur on the odd occasion. Although presenting a negligible risk to the foetus, excessive stimulation of the healing response of the mother is not desirable, since it will add to her discomfort. Provided the remedy is discontinued, or potency and dosage modified, the crisis will be of short and harmless duration. Since the likelihood of healing crisis is greater in the treatment of chronic disease, for the beginner it is advisable to avoid attempting to treat any chronic disease traits during the period of gestation and lactation. With these important matters carefully noted, you may proceed with confidence.

Concerning the matter of dietetic supplements in pregnancy, the most appropriate are brewer's yeast tablets, ii bd, and kelp (seaweed) tablets, ii bd. Both may be used from the moment pregnancy is diagnosed, they are utterly harmless, and they provide a generous supply of vitamins, and minerals. In the face of these elegant products of nature, man made 'iron pills' become a nonsense!

Where morning sickness is problematical, prescribe initially *Symphoricarpus rac.* 200 (Snowberry), 2-hourly. Should this fail, *Pulsatilla* 6, *Ipecacuanha* 6, or *Nux vomica* 6, 2-hourly. Backache often responds to *Kali. carb.* 6, 4-hourly. For constipation, if adding more roughage fails, try *Collinsonia can.* 6 (Stone-root), 4-hourly. Haemorrhoids, both in pregnancy and in general, are often soothed by the application of *Calendula* 5% cream.

Caulophyllum 30 (Blue cohosh), twice weekly (e.g. Mondays and Fridays), should be administered in all cases for the last eight weeks of gestation, in order to facilitate dilatation of the cervix in labour.

Once labour has commenced, then *Arnica* 200 and *Hypericum* 30, 2-hourly, should be given to prevent excessive bleeding, excessive bruising, and excessive pain from the perineum from stretched and damaged nerve fibres. These two remedies may be continued after delivery, bd, for several days. *Calendula* 5% cream should be applied bd to any lacerations or incisions in order to promote rapid healing. Where there is a risk of infection, administer *Pyrogen* 30, bd. Where a general anaesthetic has been administered, as for Caesarian section, and the patient is slow to recover full consciousness, administer *Opium* 30, $\frac{1}{4}$-hourly.

Cracked nipples during lactation should be treated by the application of *Calendula* 5% cream. Where lactation is discontinued, in order to prevent engorgement, prescribe *Lac caninum* 200 (Dog's milk), bd, a few doses.

20.

Works of Reference

You may study a manual of the piano all year, be put before one, and find yourself unable to play. This is why the physician should begin prescribing before embarking upon a detailed study of homoeopathic remedies and their properties. Now is the time to prepare yourself for this task, for a more thorough knowledge of remedies is necessary for the treatment of chronic disease, a matter which will shortly be at hand.

There are four main types of reference work available for study and clinical application:

1. Works that take the conventional diagnostic category as their starting point (therapeutic indices).
2. Works of *materia medica*.
3. Repertories.
4. Works concerning the relationship of remedies.

The Prescriber by Dr Clarke (Health Science Press) is probably the best example of a work in the first category. Such books are mainly of use for acute disease treatment, but do contain a certain measure of useful information with regard to chronic disease. Their weakness, however, is exposed when either we are unable to make a conventional diagnosis, or there is a grossly atypical presentation of the acute disease. That is to say, we have either no heading for the disease, or no listing of an appropriate subtype. To give you an example, a patient of mine believed he had been stung by an insect. *Apis mell.* usually deals with this problem, but he had taken it to little effect. He telephoned me for advice, and, upon close questioning, it was discovered that the lesion took the form of a bleb, an uncommon subtype. *Cantharis,* a remedy not normally thought of in the treatment of stings, though indicated in the treatment of blebs, was applied to the case with great success. Such prescribing can only be achieved by a good knowledge of the properties of remedies.

The only way to achieve a good working knowledge of the therapeutic potential of remedies is to study works of *materia medica*. These contain the following types of information, usually in great detail:

1. Symptoms, signs, and pathological changes caused by the administration of the remedy to healthy human volunteers. Such experimental administration is termed *proving,* and the documented effects constitute the *provings* of the remedy.

2. Symptoms, signs, and pathological changes caused in cases of accidental (or, perhaps, intentional) overdose or poisoning. These may be termed *accidental provings.* Together, experimental and accidental provings constitute what is termed the *pathogenesis* of the remedy. The pathogenesis, the ability of the drug to cause disease, determines, in accordance with the principle *similia similibus curentur,* its therapeutic application.

3. Symptoms, signs, pathological changes, clinical syndromes (including conventional diagnostic categories) recorded as cured by the remedy. These facts constitute the clinical corroboration of the expected potential of the remedy as deduced from the pathogenesis.

4. Comments on the *organotropic* predilections of the remedy. *Phosphorus,* for example, has a potent action on the liver.

5. Susceptible typology. This largely concerns prescription in chronic disease, and is discussed in that section.

Perhaps the best all-round work to acquire is the *Pocket Manual of Homoeopathic Materia Medica* by Dr W. Boericke. The remedies, given in their Latinized form, are listed alphabetically. Under each remedy, the accumulated pathogenetic and clinical facts are documented in sections. After an initial preamble concerning organotropic properties, and the use of the remedy in clinical syndromes, the remaining facts are classified under headings (largely anatomical) given in the following order: Mind, Head, Eyes, Ears, Nose, Face, Mouth, Stomach, Abdomen, Stool, Urine, Male, Female, Respiratory, Heart, Back, Extremities, Sleep, Fever, Skin, Modalities. Where the facts are italicized, they are to be considered as important with respect to clinical application.

The study of materia medica is always to be viewed as more important than the use of what is termed a *repertory.* The *therapeutic index* (such as *The Prescriber,* and my own initial discussions on acute disease treatment) takes its starting point as the conventional diagnosis. The *materia medica* takes the remedy. The *repertory* takes the symptom, sign, pathological change, or modality. These are usually classified in a semi-anatomical manner. Against each *rubric,* or heading, which is either a symptom, sign, pathological change, or modality, are listed a number of remedies which correspond in either their pathogeneses or known clinical effects. Thus, in one repertory, under the modality 'fat, aggravates' (concerning reaction to food), we find the following remedies listed in abbreviated form: Ars. CARB-V. *Chin.* CYC. *Fer. Grap.* PUL. Tarx. The therapeutic importance of each remedy with respect to the clinical heading is expressed by the use of an appropriate type face. Those in capitals (PULsatilla, CARBo-Veg.) are, in the opinion of the author, the major or key remedies. Then come the italicized remedies (*Chin*a, *Fer*rum met., *Grap*hites), and lastly those in plain type (Ars-enicum album). In order to find the most appropriate remedy for the case at hand, each sign, symptom, pathological change, and modality must be sought in the repertory, and the corresponding remedies carefully noted. The remedy that occurs in correspondence to either all or the majority of headings is then considered to be the most likely to cover the case, especially if it frequently appears in capitals or italics.

It is obvious that repertorization is a laborious task for the beginner, and I do not recommend it until a basic knowledge of *materia medica* has been acquired. Once, however, this has been achieved, the repertory becomes a useful clinical adjunct to remedial selection. In the case of experienced prescribers, having taken the case, they will have narrowed down the therapeutic possibilities, in most instances, to a handful of remedies. The repertory may well assist them at that point to pick the *similimum.*

Repertories are, therefore, an aid to prescription, and cannot be substituted, under any circumstances, for the study of *materia medica.* Whereas Boericke's *Pocket Manual* contains a repertory, as it does, indeed, a therapeutic index, it is not the best book for either of these. The best all-round repertory is probably *Repertory of Homoeopathic Materia Medica* by Dr J. T. Kent, especially rich in unusual ('peculiar') symptoms, but large, and unwieldy. Kent, by the way, uses thick black type instead of capitals to indicate main remedies. Perhaps better buys for the beginner would be either *A Synoptic Key of the Materia Medica* by Dr C. M. Boger (which contains a very practical repertory at the beginning), or *A Concise Repertory of Homoeopathic Medicines* by Dr S. R. Phatak.

Apart from the laborious nature of pure repertorization, there is another, and more major problem. This is the matter of clinical emphasis. Some aspects of the subjective or objective symptomatology of the case may be more important with regard to remedy selection than others. This judgement can only come with clinical experience, and a detailed knowledge of *materia medica*. Without wishing to either confuse you, or labour the point, it is not always the remedy that appears to cover the majority of the case as determined by repertorization, that is the most appropriate. It is the remedy that covers the *important* points of the case. We shall talk more of this later.

Works containing the clinical relationship of remedies should always be at hand. That by Dr Gibson Miller has already been mentioned (see page 45). You will find in this concise and practical book the following headings:

1. Remedy (that is to say, the particular remedy in relationship to which the others are considered).
2. Complements (complementary remedies).
3. Remedies that follow well.
4. Inimicals.
5. Antidotes (that is to say, those remedies that antidote the principal remedy under consideration).

A knowledge of the relationship of remedies is important after the *partial* success of an initial remedy (the first *similimum*). It is this initial remedy which we turn to in our reference work. Complementary remedies are those which frequently remove the remaining disease factors after the particular initial similimum has ceased to act. They are the best bet, so to speak. However, should the residual symptoms of the case not match the known properties of any of the listed complements, then one's attention should be turned to 'Remedies that follow well', and a selection of the most appropriate (the second *similimum*) made. The classification of remedies in this manner represents a short-cut to providing a second prescription to help complete the case. Obviously, a knowledge of *materia medica* is required to make the appropriate selection, and guess-work is certainly not to be condoned.

On many occasions, the second prescription will be made with a remedy not listed as complementary or following well. That is to say, the residual clinical picture is better matched with another remedy as deduced from the *materia medica*. In those instances, it is important to check that the second remedy is neither inimical nor antidotal in relation to the first. We must, with regard to antidotal action, check both ways in the text.

Should we fail to view the possibility of antidotal action from both sides, then we are incomplete in our appraisal. Since remedies continue to act for some time after they have been discontinued, it is obviously wise not to follow a remedy with one that has an incompatible action. Should the selection be incompatible, then it is best to find a more compatible alternative.

I have already mentioned, with reference to combined therapy, the importance of the compatibility of remedies. Where it would seem desirable to utilize combined therapies, and there is lack of information concerning the compatibility of the remedies, then it is better to use the method of alternation.

By the way, the book is not always correct; though, in its favour, I must say it errs on the side of caution. *Aconite* and *Belladonna* are listed as having an antidotal relationship, yet clinical experience demonstrates the value of the remedy *ABC!*

21.

Test Paper

There are times when it is proper to see what we have grasped. Before you embark upon the matter of the chronic diseases, you might like to test yourself with the following questions. To each question there is a single answer:

1. Which of the following techniques is *not* appropriate to the preparation of tabs. *Silicea* 6x?
   - (a) Dilution.
   - (b) Succussion.
   - (c) Trituration.
   - (d) Compression.

2. Which of the following remedies is most likely indicated in acute otitis media without perforation?
   - (a) *Mercurius sol.*
   - (b) *Arnica.*
   - (c) *Calcarea carbonica.*
   - (d) *Anthracinum.*

3. Which of the following pairs demonstrates an *inimical* relationship?
   - (a) *Aconite* and *Belladonna.*
   - (b) *Belladonna* and *Chamomilla.*
   - (c) *Oscillococcinum* and *Mercurius sol.*
   - (d) *Mercurius sol.* and *Silicea.*

4. Which remedy, prescribed in the latter months of pregnancy, is believed to assist dilatation of the cervix?
   - (a) *Lac caninum.*
   - (b) *Pulsatilla.*
   - (c) *Caulophyllum.*
   - (d) *Collinsonia.*

5. Which of the following remedies is *unlikely* to be useful in the treatment of boils?
   - (a) *Hepar sulph.*
   - (b) *Phosphorus.*
   - (c) *Belladonna.*
   - (d) *Gunpowder.*

6. Which of the following is the *inorganic* analogue of *Colocyn-*

this with respect to the treatment of colic?

  (a) *Calc. carb.*

  (b) *Mag. phos.*

  (c) *Nat. mur.*

  (d) *Kali. bich.*

7. Which of the following was the first to be proved on a healthy human volunteer?

  (a) *China.*

  (b) *Aconite.*

  (c) *Belladonna.*

  (d) *Cantharis.*

8. Which of the following remedies is a synthetic?

  (a) *Oscillococcinum.*

  (b) *China.*

  (c) *Hepar sulph.*

  (d) *Natrum mur.*

9. Which of the following statements is *untrue* with respect to the remedy *Pulsatilla?*

  (a) It is almost specific for oral thrush.

  (b) It is useful for cases of greenish catarrh.

  (c) It may be used to treat morning sickness.

  (d) It is often of service in treating measles.

10. A patient rings you to ask your advice. Her five year-old daughter has acute bronchitis, and the symptoms improved dramatically for five hours following the administration of *Antimonium tart.* 6, but have now relapsed. What is your advice?

  (a) Change the remedy.

  (b) Apply the same remedy but in a different potency.

  (c) Apply the same remedy again in the same potency.

  (d) Advise antibiotics.

11. Which of the following remedies has a direct antibiotic effect?

  (a) *Oscillococcinum.*

  (b) *Influenzinum Co.*

  (c) *Belladonna.*

  (d) None of these.

12. Which of the following remedies would you expect to have a preventative action during an epidemic of scarlet fever?

  (a) *Belladonna.*

  (b) *Myristica.*

  (c) *Spongia tosta.*

  (d) *Phosphorus.*

13. Which of the following is *not* a major remedy for the treatment of infantile croup?

   (a) *Hepar sulph.*

   (b) *Spongia tosta.*

   (c) *Aconite.*

   (d) *Pyrogen.*

14. Which of the following statements is true?

   (a) *Arsenicum album* is best prescribed in a potency of 3x.

   (b) Homoeopathic provings are carried out on people suffering from particular diseases.

   (c) Elderly people do not respond well to remedies.

   (d) *Ruta* treats non-union of fractures.

ANSWERS:

1b, 2a, 3d, 4c, 5b, 6b, 7a, 8c, 9a, 10c, 11d, 12a, 13d, 14d.

PART TWO

The Theory and Treatment
of the Chronic Diseases

22.

The Nature of Chronic Disease

The *chronic diseases* are entities of long duration. They may demonstrate their presence overtly and continuously as with osteoarthritis. Alternatively, they may *appear* to be intermittent in expression, as with recurrent migraine. However, this appearance is deceptive. Should we realize that the conventional diagnostic category (e.g. recurrent migraine) only represents a partial, and often superficial, expression of fundamental disease, then, by considering the patient as a whole, we would invariably detect the existence of disease process in phases of apparent remission.

Thus, to state a simple example, the migraine sufferer may have a background of chronic nasal catarrh, and both may be caused by a single factor, perhaps cow's milk allergy. To divide the case artificially into two different notional entities (allopathic diagnoses), migraine and catarrh, would be divorced from the reality of the situation. It would lead to the prescription of multiple palliative drugs, without any hope of anything resembling a cure. A better approach would be to remove the causative factor from the diet, the cow's milk. Furthermore, through the action of homoeopathic remedies, we may go one stage further, and eliminate the allergy to milk.

In general, therefore, when several notional chronic disease entities co-exist in the same person, it is wise, at least initially, to assume that they represent the aggregate expression of a single underlying disease factor. Our prescriptions of remedies, and our measures in general, should be targeted towards the *fundamental disease* rather than its superficial manifestations. Only in this way can we come close to the notion of *cure*.

Another wondrous illusion created by chronic disease is its apparent disappearance. The patient appears to 'grow out' of the disease. Whereas it is true that he may grow out of one notional disease entity (conventional diagnostic category), it is equally true that he may grow into another. Thus, the mucousy baby becomes an infant prone to recurrent bronchitis, an eczematous child, and then an asthmatic adult. From the homoeopathic point of view, he has grown out of nothing! Each notional phase of disease is no more than a single scene in a play written and directed by one, the fundamental disease factor. It is the latter that we must endeavour to eliminate, or at least control. This is the forte of homoeopathy.

23.
Fundamental Disease:
Genetic and Cellular

The homoeopathic concept of chronic disease is thus quite different from the allopathic. The chronic disease as it exists in a particular individual is the aggregate expression *in time and space* of symptoms, signs, and pathological changes. Those manifest in the past are considered as important for prescription as those of the present, since they may well be parts of the same disease entity. They are all to be regarded as manifestations of the same *fundamental disease* factor.

Yet, what do we surmise are these *fundamental* disease factors? In order to clarify matters, let us divide them into two types:

1. Genetic.
2. Cellular.

In our discussions, let us also consider three *modifying* elements in relation to the above:

(a) Environmental.
(b) Infective.
(c) Nutritional.

With regard to *genetic* fundamental disease, it is often erroneously thought that, by their very nature, genes are *fixed* in their mode of expression. This is obviously so with regard to many aspects of developmental anatomy within the individual, but, with regard to physiological and physiopathological processes, it is usually not the case.

In a television set the components are fixed, yet their function, the ability to show different programmes, is variable. Similarly, the components of genetic material are fixed, but their directive output is variable. The directive output may be normophysiological, or pathophysiological. Our objective in therapy is to cause a reversion from the pathological to the normal programme. We must *switch over,* so to speak, from one genetic programme to another.

Malefic (pathogenetic) genetic programmes may be either inherited or acquired. Where there is a strong family history of disease, either similar to or related to the disease of the patient, then it may be assumed that the malefic programme is of the inherited variety. Even when inherited, however, it may not necessarily be manifest from birth. It may remain as a dormant or *latent* factor for many years until the action of a modifying factor (environmental, infective, or nutritional) causes cancellation of the normophysiological programme and activation of this malefic programme. In other instances the dormancy of latency of the malefic programme is illusory.

Thus, we find that the teenager with sudden onset of asthma has, let us say, a history of catarrh since birth. In these cases, the malefic programme has always been manifest in the past, but to a minimal degree. The sudden deterioration in the patient's condition, associated with increased expression of the malefic programme, may be ascribable to the action of the aforementioned modifying factors, or exhaustion of the organs of the body, after many years of disease.

I have also made reference to the fact that malefic programmes may be acquired. Certain types of infection, such as tuberculosis or syphilis, gross nutritional problems, and prolonged exposure to harmful environments, may all lead to disturbance of genetic function. Should this not be corrected, then the malefic programme thus generated may be transmitted to the offspring in a Lamarckian fashion.

The second type of fundamental disease is the *cellular* variety. This involves general dysfunction of the cell, in the face of a normophysiological genetic programme. The messages to the components of the cell are correct, but the function of those components is deranged. This again may be due to environmental, infective, or nutritional modifying factors. Such disturbances are not inherited, but acquired. However, should they be persistent and severe, there is every risk that they will culminate in the generation of a malefic genetic programme which, as I have said, may be transmitted to the offspring. It is probable that all acquired genetic fundamental disease originates from the cellular type, by way of progression. It is also conceivable that intermediate forms of acquired fundamental disease exist between cellular dysfunction, and what we might term *the internalization* towards genetic malfunction.

It has already been stated that genetic fundamental disease may be inherited. This, indeed, is often the case. However, viewing the ancestral totality of disease within the family, it may be surmised that, at its very origins, would be the *acquisition* of a malefic genetic programme on the part of a particular ancestor. Thus, in this sense, all genetic functional disease is acquired via the phase of cellular fundamental disease, though not necessarily occurring in the lifetime of our patient, but in the lifetime of an ancestor.

These matters become of therapeutic importance when we come to the concept of *miasms* or *miasmata*. A *miasm* is a prolonged disturbance of physiology that follows infection, the infecting organism having been expelled from the body. Hence, the child who has 'never been well since ... measles'. Certain types of infection may, thus, be regarded as modifying factors with regard to the generation of fundamental disease. With regard to relatively mild infections, such as measles and whooping-cough, a corresponding miasm will not always develop. In many instances, where it does develop, it remains at the level of cellular fundamental disease for a few months, only to disappear as the result of natural healing process. However, in a few cases, the natural healing process lacks insufficient strength to remove the cellular dysfunction, and the miasm shows relentless persistence. In these instances, homoeopathic remedies are needed to remove the miasm. These generally consist of nosodes prepared from the organism responsible. Hence, a 'measles miasm', that is to say a prolonged disturbance of physiology following measles, is often nullified by the administration of a few doses of *Morbillinum* 200 (Measles nosode). This is in accordance with the Law of Similars. Prevention, of course, is better than cure, and even that small proportion of miasmic hangovers from simple childhood infections might be preventable, were homoeopathic remedies more generally applied in their treatment. *All* cases of these epidemic diseases should, in my opinion, receive the benefit of our remedies.

In the case of these common diseases of childhood, miasmic internalization from the cellular phase of fundamental disease to the genetic does not generally occur. However, with regard to more serious infective diseases, such as tuberculosis and syphilis, progression to genetic fundamental disease is a grave risk. Thus, a 'tuberculous miasm' is readily acquired, which, within a few months, passes into the more resistant genetic phase. Thus, any patient who has suffered in the past from tuberculosis, despite the removal of the infecting organism by allopathic therapy, should be suspected of having an 'ingrained' tuberculous miasm, and will require therapy with one of the group of nosodes termed the *Tuberculinums*. However, the majority of cases of tuberculous miasm that you will see in practice correspond to *acquired* genetic fundamental disease. Many cases of asthma and allergy are of this type, and a strong family history of tuberculosis rules highly in favour of this notion. It is not surprising, therefore, that the *Tuberculinum* group of remedies figure prominently in their treatment.

One other miasm warrants mention at this juncture. This is *Psora,* or the 'psoric miasm', as it is termed. This is an original Hahnemannian concept, and, perhaps, the most misunderstood in the whole field of homoeopathy. The psoric miasm results from the 'internalization' of skin disease. The skin disease may be due to fungal agents, parasitic infestation (e.g. scabies), or herpes. In some, though by no means all, instances the cutaneous infection gives rise to a profound disturbance of internal cellular function. This is made all the more likely by the use of topical agents, such as steroidal creams and sulphur ointments, which suppress the local cutaneous response, the latter being, in reality, a localizing defensive reaction on the part of the body. Thus, even though the actual skin infection may disappear, either spontaneously or through the action of topical medicines, the cellular disturbance may remain and, in turn, may progress to the phase of genetic fundamental disease.

In this manner Psora becomes an inheritable disease, and, in clinical practice, we often see its manifestations. The disease eczema is often a manifestation of inherited Psora, as might be expected; for, as a general rule with regard to any miasm, it is the 'brother' of the original disease. That is to say, it bears a pathological and organotropic similarity to the infective disease of origin. Remedies that treat Psora are termed *antipsorics,* the principal remedy being *Sulphur,* given internally.

It must be said, in all fairness, that the theory of Psora is highly controversial, even within homoeopathic circles. However, it is a strange fact that the occurrence of a transient skin rash (resembling eczema, psoriasis, herpes or scabies) is a common event during the successful homoeopathic treatment of chronic disease in general, even if the patient has no history of skin disease in the past. This could be interpreted as the symbolic representation of the original infective disease of the ancestor. Should this be so, then Hahnemann's psoric theory would be vindicated.

It is also possible for miasms to be acquired iatrogenically, through the medium of vaccination or immunization. Whereas the vaccines of diphtheria, poliomyelitis, and tetanus rarely induce miasmatic complications, the same cannot be said with regard to whooping-cough, measles or smallpox vaccine. Smallpox vaccination, in particular, especially if repeated many times in the same individual, may give rise to a particularly severe miasm, termed *Vaccinosis,* the principal remedy for which is *Thuja occidentalis* (Arbor vitae). Any individual who has had a severe reaction to smallpox vaccination in the past should be regarded as a probable suffer from Vaccinosis, and treated accordingly.

There remains to be discussed one more point, with regard to fundamental disease in general. That is, the nature of the anatomical site of fundamental disease. In which cells, or groups of cells, does it originate? The endocrine glands are, in fact, the most likely candidates for the role, whether the fundamental disease be cellular or genetic. Endocrine dysfunction leads to widespread disturbance of cellular function throughout the body. This, however, is not an easily measurable phenomenon in many cases, since the blood hormone levels may remain within the bounds of the statistically normal range. This is deceptive, for they may well be abnormal for the individual. Only in extreme cases, such as thyrotoxicosis, will there be readily discernible hormonal abnormalities.

If we assume that the endocrines are the seat of fundamental disease, then diseases such as thyrotoxicosis are to be considered as close in the chain of causation to the fundamental disease of origin. A proper understanding of individual endocrine dysfunction would lead to a better comprehension of the way in which fundamental disease exerts its action on distant sites of the body. That the endocrines become fatigued in major chronic disease of many years duration, is not, thus, entirely a secondary effect of excessive load being placed upon them. It is also due to the likely fact that they themselves are the seat of origin of the chronic disease.

24.
Modifying Factors:
Environment, Nutrition and Infection

Those which I have termed *modifying factors* may either precipitate the onset of chronic disease in their own right, or be contributory to its onset along with congenitally manifest genetic fundamental disease. As I have said, they may be infective (leading to miasmata), environmental, or nutritional. One thing they all have in common is their ability to *trigger* chronic disease, which progresses, albeit at a lesser rate, even after the offending factor has been eliminated. The residual cellular or genetic fundamental disease left in their wake maintains the chronic disease process.

Environmental and nutritional modifying factors are no less important in this respect than infective, and must be identified and corrected, where feasible. Should we fail to do so, then an apparently successful initial application of remedies will be followed by a gross relapse, since the modifying factors of disease continue to act as before. In other cases, where the modifying factors are still present and severe, no results at all will be obtained with remedies.

It is the responsibility, therefore, of *all* physicians to endeavour to identify environmental and nutritional problems in disease. Should these be largely responsible for the disease, and we are fortunate enough to intervene at an early cellular stage, where the disease is in a reversible pre-chronic mode, then rectification of these factors will lead to a complete cure without the application of remedies.

However, once the disease has progressed to a self-maintaining chronic mode, simple correction of environmental and nutritional causative factors will not effect a cure, even though such action reduces the rate of deterioration. In these circumstances, methods that include the prescription of corrective homoeopathic remedies, and special dietetic therapies, including the provision of 'supernutritional' supplements, will be required.

Environmental modifying factors include:
1. Prolonged or recurrent exposure to extremes of climate,

either within accommodation, or externally; such as excessive heat, excessive cold, or dampness.

2. Prolonged excessive psychological stress; such as that associated with overwork, financial problems, or marital discord.

3. Contact with environmental poisons; such as the prolonged inhalation of lead in the atmosphere.

4. Intra-uterine environmental problems. These, no doubt, exist, but little is known of them.

Where totally correctable, they should be eliminated. Where moderate, but not removeable, the provision of remedies over a prolonged period, in order to fortify the individual against the hostile environment, will be of service. Where the factors are severe, especially if the patient has reached the stage of mental and physical exhaustion in consequence, then there is no hope of recovery until he is removed from that environment. Remedies, allopathic drugs, all will be to no avail.

Nutritional modifying factors include:

1. Inadequate dietetic intake.

2. Inadequate intestinal absorption.

3. Excessive dietetic intake.

4. Toxic contamination of intake.

5. Intra-uterine nutritional deficiency, which may be caused by placental insufficiency, or inadequate dietetic intake by the mother.

The correction of nutritional problems is as important a part of the homoeopathic therapy of chronic disease as the prescription of remedies. This should never be forgotten. Nutritional problems in disease are commoner than many physicians would think, and, furthermore, are readily corrected. In some instances, they are the prime trigger for the chronic disease, but, more usually, they are contributory by nature. Excessive salt intake, for example, may not in its own right generate hypertension, but combine it with a genetic predisposition to this disease, and the latter will become manifest.

Inadequate dietetic intake is more common than it should be these days. It stems from plain ignorance, which is perhaps the fault of the medical profession pushing drugs rather than food, the overuse of pre-prepared convenience foods, and prolonged cooking. The commonest deficiencies, in this respect, are Zinc, the Vitamin B group, and Vitamin C.

Inadequate intestinal absorption is common in the elderly.

The gut ages, and suffers diminished function, as with other organs of the body. Vitamin B12 deficiency, which, by the way, is often missed as a diagnosis, is not the only one to be considered. Many elderly people suffer from multiple vitamin and mineral deficiencies, which stem from a combination of diminished intake and inadequate absorption. Many cases of osteo-arthritis in the elderly are associated with these nutritional problems, and receive great benefit from the provision of nutritional supplements, rather than drugs. Indeed, in general, all elderly people who present with some chronic disease should be regarded as nutritionally suspect, unless proven otherwise.

With regard to excessive intake, the worst offenders are probably salt and refined carbohydrates. These contribute to the generation of many chronic diseases found commonly in the West.

The toxic contamination of foods with artificial colouring agents (chemical dyes), artificial preservatives, insecticides, and so on, is, almost certainly, a great hazard to health. Whilst it is recognized that many hyperactive children are, in fact, the victims of such poisoning, especially with chemical dyes, it is not generally realized that other more insidious diseases may stem from these toxins. It is right that we exclude them as best we can from our diets.

The contamination of food with aluminium presents a problem to a small percentage of the population. These people suffer from so-called *aluminium sensitivity,* and, for them, aluminium is to be regarded as a most toxic ingested substance. Signs of aluminium toxicity include:
1. Great tendency to constipation, in the face of a good intake of dietary fibre.
2. Flatulence.
3. Severe muscular cramps.
4. General disturbance of endocrine function.
5. Fluid retention.

Proof of the condition, and cure are made by total removal of disease following total exclusion of ingested aluminium.

For practical reasons *food allergy* may be regarded as a form of ingested toxicity, for, to those who suffer from the condition, the offending foods, to all intents and purposes, function as toxins. However, food allergy, in itself, cannot be regarded as a fundamental disease in its own right. It is part of a general allergic problem, the fundamental genetic cause of which should be corrected with homoeopathic remedies. Nevertheless, since any toxic reaction may interfere with the action of remedies, it is wise to identify the offending foods, and exclude them totally whilst the remedies are acting. In this way, treatment failures will be less frequent, and most patients will then be rendered insensitive to the originally allergenic food.

Nutritional deficiencies in pregnant or lactating women, and, therefore, in the foetus or infant, are often preventable by prescribing adequate quantities of brewer's yeast and kelp (4-6 tablets a day of each). These may be prescribed with impunity from the moment that pregnancy is diagnosed, and are perfectly safe in the first trimester. They are vastly preferable to the administration of man-made iron pills and folic acid tablets. They are very cheap, well tolerated, easily absorbed, and together contain more elements than the artificial prescriptions usually issued.

25.

The Concept of Cure

The first paragraph of Hahnemann's *Organon* reads: 'The physician's high and *only* mission is to restore the sick to health, to cure, as it is termed'.

Yet, what do we mean by the word cure? And this is no mere semantic riddle, but a matter of grave importance to the patient, for it concerns his prognosis. It also affects the physician himself, for it determines the limits of his therapeutic capabilities.

Taken at face value, the word *cure* would seem to convey total eradication of disease with no recurrence. Yet, there is a philosophical problem inherent in such an interpretation. For, the absolute eradication of all disease in a particular individual would lead to immortality. Since not one person to date, to the best of my knowledge, has achieved a state of immortality, it would seem probable that no physician may lay claim to the ability to cure all disease *in toto*.

The word *cure,* therefore, must be taken to mean something less than it would imply on face value. It is, so to speak, a relative term. In terms of the theory of chronic diseases which I have set before you, we are obliged to assess the levels of cure that are practically attainable.

The first, and most important thing to be said is with regard to the modifying factors; those matters of infection, environment, and nutrition which have a causative role in the onset of chronic disease. No case can be considered as stable if we do not identify these factors, and ensure that they are no longer present. Where a simple modifying factor, such as grief from the loss of a close relative, has induced the disease, then the prognosis is often excellent, for the initiating element of the disease exists in the past, and the physician has only the aftermath with which to contend. Even then, the patient must be warned that a similar course of events is likely to occur, should he receive another similar emotional shock. Furthermore, he must be advised to seek immediate homoeopathic advice in this eventuality, in order to prevent recrudescence of chronic disease.

In other cases, the modifying factor is irremoveable. For financial reasons, the patient may be obliged to remain living in a boggy, damp area, this inimical environment to be held responsible for the onset of his arthritis. In such cases, long-term stabilizing remedies may be required to fortify him against his environment. Thus, such a patient may be compelled to take intermittent doses of the remedy *Natrum sulph.* (Sodium sulphate) for many years to oppose the effects of cold and damp.

In other instances, the modifying factors are highly speculative, or unknown. Hence, we cannot know whether they are still present. Our prognosis must, therefore, be guarded.

Let us now consider the notion of cure in relation to fundamental disease itself, genetic or cellular. Genetic fundamental disease, as I have said, is the manifestation of a pathogenetic or malefic programme. It is probable that such programmes, be they inherited or acquired, cannot be annihilated, but rather are rendered dormant or latent by therapeutic action. The concept of cure, therefore, in relation to genetic fundamental disease is, at the best, to render it permanently dormant. We must always bear in mind this fact that the malefic programme remains as a potential of the genetic material, and may become reactivated through the activity of one or more modifying factors. Diseases of well-defined genetic origin, where there is a strong familial trait, must be considered in this manner.

By contrast, simple cellular fundamental disease, where, by definition, there is no genetic malfunction, is, in its early stages, totally correctable. However, it too may recur if the body is exposed to an appropriate modifying factor. The measles miasm is an example of a cellular fundamental disease that is totally removeable, and not likely to recur. For, once it has been removed by remedies, the natural immunity to reinfection with the same organism usually guarantees that it will not happen again,

Of course, genetic fundamental disease must manifest itself as cellular dysfunction. Whether this be such a secondary phenomenon of genetic origin, or a primary cellular fundamental disease, it is inevitable that prolonged dysfunction of either sort will eventually lead to permanent irreversible anatomical and physiological changes. Thus, let us now consider the notion of cure as it applies to the level of cellular dysfunction in general, whether primary or secondary.

As has been stated with regard to primary cellular fundamental disease, cellular dysfunction in general is totally reversible in its initial stages. There is merely a disturbance of the function of the cell. This emphasizes the importance of recognizing the appearance of chronic disease in its earliest phase. Thus, early homoeopathic intervention in the case of an infant with mild chronic nasal catarrh will completely normalize cellular function, and prevent its development into a more serious disease, such as serous otitis media, asthma, and so on. If we fail to recognize these subtle changes as being premonitory with regard to the development of more serious disease in later years, then we do the patient a disservice.

Left unchecked, the reversible mode of cellular dysfunction progresses to anatomical disorganization, both of the cell and the arrangement of cells within the organs of the body, with further disturbance of the physiology. Even so, appropriate intervention may arrest this progression, and, in some cases, a certain degree of anatomical recovery will be possible. Hence, it is not unknown in the homoeopathic therapy of osteoarthritis for areas of bony overgrowth to reduce in size. However, once anatomical changes have occurred, the likelihood of *total* return to normality is slim, and this more so when the changes are gross. Nevertheless, it is often surprising the degree to which anatomical reversal is possible through the action of remedies. I have personally witnessed the disappearance of large and calcified cysts, and Dupuytren's contractures under the influence of the remedy *Calcarea fluorica* (Calcium fluoride).

Thus, the definition of *cure* is not a simple matter, for contained in this word is a spectrum of meanings. That all disease can be totally eradicated in the individual, as I have said, is an impossibility. Yet, homoeopathy, with its ability to subdue fundamental disease (genetic or cellular), to identify modifying factors, and eliminate them where possible, to reverse anatomical changes, to a certain degree, and to act with safety, must constitute, in all reason, a *curative* system of medicine.

26.
The Complexity of Chronic Disease

From the moment of conception, the individual is subject to the action of modifying factors. Although we classify these factors into environmental, infective, and nutritional categories, they are all, in reality, of exogenous or environmental nature. As we pass through life, the effects of these exogenous factors are heaped upon our bodies. Thus, the structure of disease in the child is generally less complex than that in the adult, for he has experienced less environmental modification. As might be expected, therefore, the rectification of chronic disease in the child is a simpler task than in the case of the adult. This is where, ideally, we should commence therapy. Furthermore, the whole task of therapy is made considerably simpler by the fact that little or no anatomical change has occurred in the child, the disease essentially being one of cellular dysfunction at a reversible stage. Additionally, it must be stated that healing is always achieved more swiftly in bodies undergoing growth. Growth promotes healing, so to speak.

I have stated, with regard to the coexistence of several notional chronic disease entities within the same individual, that it is ideal, at least initially, to consider that they correspond to a single genetic or cellular fundamental disease factor. That is to say, from the therapeutic point of view, it is judicious to institute a simple programme to treat the totality of the disease, rather than to attempt to treat each end-product of disease. Such treatment might entail removal of nutritional and environmental modifying factors and the application of a *single* homoeopathic remedy to rectify the fundamental disease. Such a remedy is termed the *constitutional* remedy, and the way in which it is selected is discussed later.

Indeed, this simple approach will generally be highly successful in the case of the child, for his structure of disease is usally simple and uncomplicated. In the case of the adult, however, disease is generally more complex, with the coexistence of multiple fundamental disease factors. Even where disease is still at the stage of reversible cellular dysfunction, the adult may require the application of a *succession* of constitutional remedies to rectify the complex basis of his problems. Even broad-acting *polychrests,* such as *Sulphur,* may not have enough range to cover the complexity of the fundamental disease. Even so, it must be admitted that the practitioner often meets cases of children who, because of severe exogenous activity, or the inheritance of multiple malefic genetic programmes, present as much as a therapeutic problem as the adult.

You are now ready to enter the realms of practical chronic disease therapy. In the discussions that follow, you will learn how to prescribe remedies; but what you must learn first is how to adjust nutrition. Much good work is done with nutritional changes alone.

27.
A Sensible Basic Diet

We shall be coming to the matter of special diets used in the treatment of chronic disease in due course. Most special diets are, in fact, modifications of what might be termed a *sensible basic diet*. Even where special diets are not indicated, your patients, and you yourself, moreover, should follow the basic principles given below, as closely as possible. This diet is not only contributory to cure in many cases, but also preventative:

1. The consumption of *white flour* is disallowed. White flour usually contains numerous chemical additives, which may be harmful. Deprived of wheat husk (bran), it is not only digested too rapidly, resulting in an excessive load on the insulin-producing cells, but also then lacks a material which is known to maintain the health of the gut. *Wholemeal flour* incurs none of these disadvantages.

2. Foods containing *artificial colouring agents* and *artificial preservatives* are disallowed. These substances are potentially toxic, and their exclusion is not merely indicated in the case of hyperactive children. Many foods these days contain harmful dyes, including processed peas, kippers, ice-cream, and many sweet drinks. With regard to preservatives, vinegar in small quantities is harmless and allowable. Since many manufacturers are now marketing foods totally free of these substances, there would seem little commercial excuse for using them at all. For this perpetuation of harmful absurdity, we must blame our illustrious governments and their impotent medical advisers.

3. *Sugar* intake should be kept to a minimum. Excessive intake of sugar has been implicated in the development of diabetes and cardiovascular disease. It also tends to aggravate certain skin diseases, such as eczema and acne. Brown sugar is probably only marginally better than white, and honey is the best alternative; though even excesses of honey can be harmful.

4. *Animal fat* intake should be kept to a minimum. This includes: lard, fatty meat (particularly pork and lamb), eggs, butter, cream. This is also implicated in the development of cardiovascular disease. One egg a day is probably safe and beneficial.

5. Excessive intake of *fried foods* should be avoided, even if the cooking agent is a vegetable oil. Vegetable oils are vastly preferable to animal fats, but all fats and oils are highly calorific. They tend, therefore, to promote obesity. Additionally, all fats and oils, taken to excess, place an unwarranted load on the biliary system.

6. *Salt* intake should be kept at a low level, except for those who live or work in excessively hot environments. Prolonged, excessive intake of salt places a great strain on the renal mechanism, and is contributory to the development and maintenance of hypertension. A salt substitute, containing potassium chloride, is available for those who do not dislike its slightly bitter taste.

7. Excesses of *alcohol* should be avoided. It is better for your liver to drink in fits and starts, than to drink steadily and regularly. In this way, it has a chance to recover between drinking sessions.

8. The consumption of *grain husk (bran)* is to be encouraged. In those who consume a reasonable amount of whole-grains in their regular diet, such as wholemeal bread and brown rice, the provision of extra dietary fibre may be unnecessary. In those whose grain intake is small, and those who suffer from constipation or diverticulitis, the addition of extra bran is often advisable. For adults, approximately one or two tablespoonsful of bran should be taken daily. Those who are gluten sensitive should avoid the use of wheat bran, since it may be contaminated with small quantities of this substance.

Bran is not only a mechanical aid to the function of the gut, but also mops up toxins in the latter, rather like a sponge. However, there is a small percentage of patients who become excessively flatulent and generally unwell on a high fibre diet. These people require low fibre diets, with the exclusion of bran, and minimization of their whole-grain intake. Some suffer this so badly that they must have bread made from *additive-free* white flour, which is obtainable, but with some difficulty. Patients who make a sudden change from a poor diet to a wholefood diet, tend to experience flatulence and looseness of motions initially. This generally wears off in a few weeks. Should it be a persistent problem, however, their bran or whole-grain intake must be reduced.

9. The consumption of a good quantity of fresh *fruit* and *vegetables* is to be encouraged. About fifty per cent by volume of the vegetables should be eaten raw, and the remainder only

lightly cooked. They may be boiled for a short time, steamed, or stir-fried in the Chinese fashion, but the oil should not be allowed to smoke, for this may produce carcinogens. Similarly, excessive intake of barbecued food is hazardous. Prolonged cooking of vegetables reduces their vitamin and mineral content. Where fresh vegetables are not readily obtainable, the frozen variety are the next best thing. Canned vegetables are definitely at the bottom of the list of preferences.

You are avised to compose a short dietetic guide-sheet for the use of your patients, based on the above concepts. This will enable them to study the principles in their own time, rather than yours. Whereas such words as 'excessive' and 'minimum' may seem vague, clinical experience with diet sheets worded in this manner demonstrates that they are, in actual practice, readily comprehensible to the majority of patients. That is to say, humans have sufficient intelligence and intuitive understanding of their own constitutional structure to interpret these dietetic statements in the manner most beneficially suited to them. This statement not only applies to adults, but also to many children of eight years or more. It is surprising how children can be, in some cases, more conscientious over dietetic measures than many adults.

We now pass to the matter of special diets, which, as I have said, are generally modifications of the basic diet.

28.

Constipation

Constipation may be defined as the passage of motions less than once daily, or the necessity to strain at stool. Constipation is not only uncomfortable for the patient, but also leads to the reabsorption of faecal toxins. In consequence, the patient will feel generally unwell.

Simple dietetic rectification with the measures of the basic diet, including additional bran, will often correct this disorder. Should this fail, then prunes, or raw mushrooms (2 oz/60g twice daily) may be added to the diet. Difficult cases often respond to figs, or occasional doses of syrup of figs. In most obstinate cases, the use of potent laxatives is not to be encouraged, but glycerine suppositories are acceptable, since their effect is a purely mechanical one.

Patients who suffer from haemorrhoids should never allow themselves to become constipated.

29.

Indigestion

Patients who suffer from *indigestion*, whatever the cause, should avoid the following:

1. Citrus fruits.
2. Lettuce.
3. Tomato.
4. Cucumber.
5. Fruit skins (all fruit should be peeled).
6. Highly spiced foods.
7. Neat spirits.
8. Large amounts of bread.

Since cabbage has a beneficial effect on the stomach, sufferers from indigestion are advised to eat raw grated cabbage (red, white or green) on a daily basis, with a little olive oil dressing. Cabbage can be a most potent healer of peptic ulcers, and olive oil exerts some protective function itself.

Alfalfa has a similar beneficial action. It may be taken in the form of young sprouts, which are very easily produced from seed, or in the form of compressed tablets of alfalfa. Whereas the flavour of the young sprouts is excellent, that of the tablets is not to the taste of most. These should be swallowed, therefore, a satisfactory quantity being ii tid after meals.

A tea made by infusing one or two split green cardamom pods in a cup of weak ordinary tea has a soothing action on the stomach, and may be used regularly before or after meals. Green cardamoms are readily obtainable from Asian stores. When splitting the pods, do not remove the core of seeds.

Patients suffering from disease of the *gall-bladder* require a diet very low in both animal fats and vegetable oils. It is better if they can be persuaded to abstain from meat altogether, and to minimize their intake of dairy products. Non-oily fish, such as cod and haddock, may be eaten freely, but these, of course, should not be fried in oil. Oily fish, such as mackerel and herring, are disallowed.

Patients who suffer from simple excessive *lower abdominal flatulence* are advised to reduce their consumption of peas, beans, lentils, and members of the cabbage family (cabbage, Brussels sprouts, etc.).

30.

Diet in Arthritis

Patients suffering from *arthritic* conditions, especially if there is a well-defined inflammatory component, often benefit from the following:

1. The exclusion, or reduction, of pork, beef, veal, lamb, game and dark poultry meat.

2. The consumption of 1-2 pints ($\frac{1}{2}$-1 litre) of fruit juice or vegetable juice daily, taken in divided quantities.

Fruit juices of high organic acidity, such as orange or grapefruit, may not be tolerated in large quantities, since they may be irritant to the stomach. Juices such as tomato and pineapple are better tolerated in large quantity. Fruit juices should always be of the unsweetened type, and should not contain preservatives.

The same diet is of value in the treatment of some localized musculo-skeletal problems, such as sciatica and lumbago.

Nutritional deficiency must always be considered as a possibility in the elderly, and dietetic supplements may be required, this matter being discussed in due course. Food allergy and aluminium sensitivity are implicated in a small percentage of cases of inflammatory arthritis, and these too will be discussed.

31.

Hypoglycaemia

Hypoglycaemia is a condition which is becoming alarmingly common in modern society. It is a condition basically associated with prolonged or recurrent psychological stress. The busy housewife and the overworked businessman are equally at risk of developing this disease. A diagnosis of hypoglycaemia in a very relaxed person is unlikely.

The mechanism of this condition is fairly simple in principle. Psychological stress sensitizes the insulin-release mechanism of the pancreas, so that excessive quantities of insulin are secreted in response to glucose entering the blood-stream from the intestine. This results in a fall of blood sugar. The greater the quantity of glucose coming from the gut, the more exaggerated is the pancreatic response.

The object of therapy, therefore, is to reduce radically the dietary intake of sugars, and carbohydrates that are rapidly converted to sugar.

The symptoms of hypoglycaemia may include any of the following:

1. Excessive hunger, especially if a meal is delayed, even for a short time.
2. Shaking and trembling, especially before mealtimes, or if meals are delayed.
3. Relief of symptoms by eating.
4. Attacks of faintness or dizziness.
5. Migraine, especially if atypical, with hunger during the attack, and some relief with eating.
6. Craving for sweet things.
7. Neurotic behaviour, with tendency to aggression.
8. Tendency to alcoholism, or addiction to nicotine.
9. Excessive sweating.
10. Rapid fatigue
11. Diarrhoea.
12. Palpitations.

All symptoms tend to remit with exercise, or the removal of the cause of the stress. If the cause of the stress cannot be removed, then the *hypoglycaemic diet* given below will produce great improvement. The use of relaxation techniques, such as yoga, regular exercise, and the beneficial application of homoeopathic remedies should not be forgotten as being complementary to the dietetic regime. The diagnosis of hypoglycaemia is confirmed by a positive response to the diet. Laboratory confirmation of the condition involves a five-hour glucose tolerance test, which is generally unnecessary, since both diagnosis and 'cure' can be effected by simple dietetic rectification. Undoubtedly, a large number of apparently psycho-neurotic patients receive antidepressant and tranquillizing drugs for years, when the mainstay of their treatment should be of a dietetic nature.

The special diet is as follows:

DISALLOWED	ALLOWED
Sugar	Meat
Honey	Fish
Cakes	Wholemeal flour
Biscuits	Brown rice
White wheat flour	Buckwheat
Cornflour	Millet
Marmalade and jam	Brown pasta
Porridge	Lightly cooked root vegetables
Well-cooked root vegetables	Lightly cooked peas
Well-cooked peas	Lightly cooked beans
Well-cooked beans	All raw vegetables
Cooked potatoes	Fresh fruits
Squash or fizzy drinks	Unsweetened fruit juice
White rice	Canned unsweetened fruit
Canned sweetened fruit	Dried fruit (in moderation)
Alcohol	Mushrooms
Large amounts of milk	Muesli (unsweetened)
and milk products	Nuts
Canned vegetables.	A little milk, and milk products
	in moderation
	Eggs.

This is the diet needed at the outset. However, it may be subject to modification *by the physician*. In many cases we find considerable relief of the presenting symptoms, but the patients complain of general weakness. In such circumstances, we have reduced the glucogenic content of the diet by too great a degree.

The addition of, say, one baked potato daily will often correct this problem.

Patients also vary considerably in the severity of their hypoglycaemia, and some will tolerate additions to the diet that would be catastrophic for others. If alcohol is to be gingerly added back to the diet, then it is best to choose a low-alcohol (about 8 per cent by volume) dry or medium-dry wine. German wines often conform to these requirements. Obviously, the diet I have suggested does not mention every possible food. You should be able to answer patients' questions with regard to any not mentioned, bearing in mind the principles of the diet.

After commencing the special diet, some patients may experience hunger between normal mealtimes. They should be advised to take snacks of acceptable foods (e.g. wholemeal bread, raw vegetables) as often as necessary. As therapy continues, the necessity for such measures diminishes. You will find that many patients lose weight initially on this diet, but this generally plateaus out after a month or so. This is obviously a boon to the overweight patient, but may be a source of alarm to the thin one, who may need reassurance on the matter.

As a matter of interest, many women suffering from *premenstrual tension* show symptoms of hypoglycaemia in the premenstrual phase, though not necessarily during the rest of the cycle. These women should be advised to follow the hypoglycaemic diet in the premenstrual phase, or, more stringently, a diet consisting of fresh fruit and brown rice alone.

32.
The Grape Cure

The *grape cure* is a dietetic technique designed to cleanse the body of toxins (endogenous and exogenous), and to promote healing in cases of chronic disease. Essentially, this consists of the total exclusion of all foods other than well-washed, well-ripened grapes. The only drink allowed is pure spring-water, which may readily be obtained in bottles from supermarkets (Shropshire water, Malvern water, etc.). It is to be emphasized that the grapes must be sweet, rather than sour, for sour grapes are intolerable in large quantities. The quantity of grapes to be consumed each day should not be less than $1\frac{1}{2}$ lbs ($\frac{3}{4}$ kilo), and about one third of the skins and pips should be swallowed to prevent constipation.

First attempts at the grape cure should not exceed three days in duration. By the third day, most people will experience a 'healing crisis', consisting of headache, malaise, exaggeration of current symptoms of disease, or fatigue. This should be explained to the patient prior to therapy so that he is not caught unawares. Following discontinuation of the grape cure, the patient experiences a 'healing phase', when general well-being improves to a level higher than that prior to the treatment.

Should the response to this dietetic therapy be satisfactory, and the patient willing, the grape cure may be repeated each month, for three days. In some cases it is permissible to extend the treatment to a week or more.

Because of the ability to detoxify the body with great rapidity, the grape cure is particularly useful where we wish to abandon the use of conventional drugs as swiftly as possible. Whereas in certain cases of serious disease, such as asthma, it would be unwise to discontinue conventional drugs abruptly, there are some situations when it is advisable. For example, in the case of the patient on long-term tranquillizers or antidepressants, where the original disease has long since disappeared, only to be replaced by an iatrogenic disease, viz. physical and mental drug dependency. The patient is then taking the drug essentially to prevent withdrawal symptoms. As soon as the drug is withdrawn, the grape cure must be commenced. In a like manner, the grape cure is of service in the management of allergic drug response. It has also been used, with some success, in the treatment of cancer, a disease in which the patient has the accumulation of endogenous toxins to a great degree.

Since the grape cure is a potent instrument of healing, it should not be used for children, the severely malnourished (except in cancer), or in pregnancy and lactation. It is also unsuitable for diabetics on insulin, for they will have difficulty in judging their requirements of this substance. It should also be used with caution in elderly patients, or those who suffer from serious heart disease, for fear of putting an excessive load upon them in the crisis phase.

33.

Veganism and Vegetarianism

Veganism involves the total exclusion of *all* animal products from the diet; meat, fish, milk, eggs, and so on. In general, despite assertions to the contrary, veganism is a culturally or ethically determined dietetic system, rather than a therapeutic method. With regard to its preventative claims, it seems to have no advantage over lacto-vegetarianism or traditional semi-vegetarianism (the exclusion of only meat and poultry). Furthermore, vegans are always in danger of developing Vitamin B^{12} deficiency, which may be prevented by taking suitable quantities of vegan oral B^{12} supplement. This matter should always be contemplated when you interview a vegan patient. One thing that you are not entitled to do is to tread on the ethical toes of the patient.

However, there is one particular disease that may be affected beneficially by the institution of a vegan diet. That is *psoriasis*. Provided the patient is willing, and most are, they should be kept on a vegan diet for several months. This, plus the administration of appropriate homoeopathic remedies, brings relief to many sufferers. Whilst the patient follows this strict diet, oral B^{12} supplement should be taken, 25-50 microgrammes daily. As improvement occurs, some animal products, such as fish, may be re-introduced if the patient is becoming bored with the system.

34.

Aluminium Sensitivity

Patients believed to be suffering from *aluminium sensitivity* (see section 24) should follow the following regime in order to exclude ingested aluminium. A favourable result tends to imply a correct diagnosis:

1. The consumption of foods cooked, prepared, or stored in aluminium vessels is disallowed.

2. Cooking pans made of enamelled steel, stainless steel, or iron are acceptable.

3. Foods wrapped in aluminium foil are disallowed.

4. Fruit-juices contained in foil-lined cartons are disallowed.

5. Bottled fruit-juices are acceptable.

6. Canned foods are disallowed. Also canned or kegged drinks.

7. Frozen foods, where the fresh varieties are unavailable, are generally permissible.

8. Caution should be observed when eating out, with regard to the aluminium content of food or drink.

9. In some cases, the patients appear to be sensitive to tap-water. This may be due to its aluminium content. It may be necessary, therefore, to place them on bottled spring-water.

Once the patient has improved on this regime, he is sometimes committed to it indefinitely, although, in some cases, the application of constitutional remedies eliminates or reduces the sensitivity. Obviously, whilst the patient eats and drinks at home, there is little problem, once he has adjusted to the procedure. However, the principal disadvantage of aluminium sensitivity is with regard to eating out, whether as a guest of a friend, or in a restaurant. In the former case, it may be a positive embarrassment to ask about the nature of the hostess's cooking pots.

Fortunately, it is often possible to antidote the ill-effects of occasional episodes of aluminium ingestion with homoeopathic remedies. Thus, before going to eat out, the patient should take a single dose of either *Alumina* 6x (Aluminium oxide), or *Cuprum met.* 10x (Copper) mixed with *Sulphur* 10x. The same remedy should be repeated upon returning home, and a few subsequent doses given 12-hourly thereafter. Only in very mild cases of aluminium sensitivity are these remedies of any value in the long-term prevention of the disorder without dietetic modification. Exclusion of the offending substance is the mainstay of therapy in the majority of cases.

35.

Food Allergy

Food allergy is a diagnosis commonly missed with regard to chronic disease. In the case of the patient who explodes in urticaria after eating strawberries, and this occurs within a short time after their ingestion, the diagnosis is obvious, and few physicians, let alone patients, would miss it. This type of food allergy, therefore, is seldom a causative factor in chronic disease, for the offending agent is easily identified and excluded totally from the diet, this often being done without professional advice. In most cases, however, the manifestations of food allergy are more insidious than this. Let us consider, therefore, those pointers which should lead the physician to suspect the possibility of the presence of food allergy:

1. A tingling feeling of the tongue, or feeling of constriction in the throat, upon the ingestion of certain foods. This is an immediate reaction, and uncommon.

2. A definite time interval between the onset of recurrent acute symptoms and the ingestion of certain foods, e.g. headache always comes on six hours after drinking beer in moderation. The time interval may be anything from a few minutes in some cases, to a day or so in others. The longer the time interval, the less likely is the patient to associate the symptoms with a particular allergen.

3. Intense dislike of certain foods, especially since childhood, without tangible reason being offered by the patient. This may constitute intuitive knowledge of allergenic foods, but more likely is the subconscious aftermath of a previous conscious experience of food reaction, long since forgotten.

4. Intense craving for certain foods. This is rather like drug addiction. A regular intake of the offending food is necessary to prevent withdrawal symptoms.

5. A child is perfectly well whilst breast-fed, but falls ill upon weaning.

6. A strong family history of food allergy, or allergies in general, or diseases such as asthma and migraine.

7. The presence of other allergies in the patient. Thus, food

allergy may be associated with inhalant or contact allergy. Unlike hay-fever, the manifestations of food allergy are perennial rather than seasonal.

8. Certain types of disease *may* be associated with food allergy. The occurrence of more than one diagnostic entity, within the *total* history of the patient from birth, is greater evidence of food allergy:

(a) Recurrent migraine. However, if the attacks are very infrequent (e.g. three times per year), food allergy as a cause is unlikely. Similarly, it is an unlikely cause in cases of periodic migraine of women, where the attacks occur regularly, with a well-defined periodicity of two to four weeks.

(b) Recurrent non-migrainous headaches.

(c) Chronic nasal catarrh or obstruction.

(d) Chronic sinusitis.

(e) Snuffly babies.

(f) Chronic eustachian catarrh.

(g) Serous otitis media.

(h) Recurrent migrainous neuralgia of the face.

(i) Persistent diarrhoea, or looseness of the bowels.

(j) Crohn's disease.

(k) Ulcerative colitis.

(l) Recurrent urticaria.

(m) Asthma. Here, food allergy and inhalant allergy often coexist.

(n) Eczema. Especially, if it appears upon weaning.

(o) Multiple sclerosis (rarely).

(p) Inflammatory arthritis (rarely).

(q) Hyperactivity and unco-operative behaviour of childhood.

The greater the number of these points present in a particular case, the more likely the diagnosis of food allergy is positive. Since it warrants restatement, you must take into consideration the *total* history of the patient from birth. Having considered that food allergy is a definite possibility, the next thing to be determined is the identity of the offending foods. I say 'foods' rather than 'food', for, in general, most cases exhibit allergy to more than one, although one particular food may be dominant in its effects. We may determine the identity of those foods in any of the following ways:

1. Food allergy tests. These include:

(a) Skin testing. Very unreliable.

(b) Laboratory blood test. Reliable, but may be expensive, and not readily available.

(c) Pulse test. Changes in the pulse are observed when solutions of offending foods are introduced sublingually. Requires great skill for interpretation, and many false positives are obtained.

(d) Muscular kinesthetic test. Changes in muscle tone are observed when solutions of offending foods are introduced sublingually. Requires great skill for interpreation.

2. On the basis of the history.

3. Exclusion diets (diagnostic).

From the point of view of general practice, methods 2. and 3. are most appropriate to the identification of allergenic foods. Indeed, it is practical to discuss them conjointly.

Exclusion diets are designed to demonstrate improvement of the patient in association with removal of one or more elements from the general diet. The general diet from which the exclusions are made should conform to the principles of the *sensible basic diet* discussed previously. There are various ways in carrying out exclusions, but I shall outline one for which I have a personal preference, since it is both simple and effective. This is based on the relative probability of foods being allergenic in any particular case, as determined by clinical experience.

Consider the following groups, given in descending order of probable allergenicity with respect to any case (Group A, most likely; Group D, least likely):

GROUP A*	GROUP B	GROUP C	GROUP D
Suspect foods as determined by case history.	Cow's milk. Wheat. Malt. Chocolate	Citrus fruits. Corn (maize). Yeast. Tomato.	Beef. Pork. Lamb.

*Group A may include elements of B, C or D.

Exclusion diets should always be carried out for approximately one month before the results are assessed. Whereas cases showing little or no organic change (e.g. simple migraine) often show positive results in a week or two, those where anatomical change has occurred to a significant degree (e.g. chronic sinusitis) may take up to a month, and sometimes longer, to show any noticeable improvement.

For the purpose of speedy analysis, each group is initially excluded *in toto,* in accordance with the following programme:

1. *First month.* Place patient on the basic sensible diet.

Simultaneously, exclude Group A (if there is no Group A, then commence with Group B exclusions, and adjust the directions given hereafter accordingly). If, at the end of one month, the results are excellent, continue the regime for one further month to stabilize the case. Maintain the sensible basic diet. Then, if several foods have been excluded, reintroduce them at the rate of one per month, until relapse occurs. Next, re-exclude the offending food for one month, in order to restabilize the case. Any of the remaining foods of the group may then be reintroduced, at the rate of one per month, and their allergenicity determined in a similar manner. If the excellent results of the first month are maintained, despite reinclusion of *all* foods of Group A, then it must be assumed that the improvement has occurred due to placing the patient on the basic sensible diet. In this instance, the patient may be suffering from allergy to food additives, or hypoglycaemia.

2. If the results of Group A exclusion are negative, for the *second month* reintroduce Group A, and exclude Group B. Remember to maintain the basic sensible diet. Always exclude Group B *in toto,* unless one or more foods have been represented in Group A, and tested accordingly in the first month. These foods need not be excluded.

If the results of Group A exclusion in the first month are partial or equivocal, for the second month you must exclude both Groups A and B, whilst maintaining the basic sensible diet.

Excellent results warrant the reintroduction of individual foods on a monthly basis, as described above, to determine those allergenic to the patient.

If the results of Group B exclusion alone are negative, reintroduce Group B, and exclude Group C for the *third month.* Maintain the basic diet. If partially successful or equivocal, exclude both Groups B and C.

If the results of excluding both Groups A and B are no better than with the exclusion of A alone, then reintroduce Group B, and continue with the exclusion of both A and C.

If the results of excluding both Groups A and B are marginally better than with the exclusion of A alone, proceed with the exclusion of Groups A, B, and C.

Excellent results warrant the reinclusion system described previously. You should be able now to deduce what to do, if the results are partial or equivocal.

But what if we reach Group D exclusion, and the patient has not improved? There are two possibilities. Firstly, that the patient is allergic to a food not on our list, in which case, should this be a definite possibility, the patient should be referred to a physician specializing in food allergy. Secondly, and perhaps more likely in most cases, the patient does not exhibit food allergy. After all, most patients who suffer from food allergy usually have intolerance of more than one food, and, in most cases, at least one of the offenders will have been revealed by our simple programme, the exclusion of which produces partial results at least.

Since the majority of cases of food allergy largely fall within Groups A and B, it is often but a simple matter to sort out the relevant allergens, or the major allergens at least.

With regard to cow's milk, it must be remembered to exclude all its products. These include butter, cheese, yogurt, and whey. The latter is incorporated in many margarines, and the patient must be advised to obtain a vegan margarine (free of animal products), readily available from health food stores. Goat's milk and its products may be substituted for those of the cow in most cases, since allergy to goat's milk is rare. Alternatively, soya milk may be used. Allergy to soya milk is also a rarity.

Allergy to wheat is fairly common, but may be part of a larger sensitivity to gluten. Gluten sensitivity is not merely seen in relation to coeliac disease, and lesser sensitivity may be protean in its manifestations. Where wheat exclusion has produced partial improvement of the patient, and no other allergens have been found, it is wise to consider the subsequent exclusion of all foods that contain gluten for one month. This is essentially a diet that contains no common grains, but rice, which is gluten-free, is allowable.

Malt exclusion tends to be an enormous problem for the patient, or those who shop for him, since it is used as a flavouring in so many foods (e.g. bread, breakfast cereals, beer). Great vigilance is required when inspecting lists of ingredients as quoted by the manufacturers.

When carrying out exclusion diets, it is wise to note that the removal of potent allergens *may* produce withdrawal symptoms, or 'healing crisis', as it is termed. This is akin to the concept of withdrawal with respect of other toxic substances, such as morphine. Thus, the migraine sufferer may experience increased severity and frequency of his complaint, following withdrawal of the toxic food. This is always followed by an improvement phase (healing phase). Eczema, in a similar manner, may temporarily worsen. Patients should always be informed of this possibility, in order to prevent alarm, should the crisis occur. Generally speaking, most healing crises occur and peak within one or two weeks of commencing the exclusion. By the time the patient is reviewed at one month, he is usually in the healing phase.

The deductions made from the *diagnostic* exclusion diet will obviously form the basis of the *therapeutic* exclusion diet. Partial results with either diagnostic or therapeutic exclusion diets may be attributable to various factors:

(a) Failure of the patient to carry out total exclusion. This may be due to reluctance, or unintentional ingestion of offending foods. It is not generally known, for example, that white flour contains cow's milk.

(b) Failure of the physician to detect all relevant ingested allergens.

(c) The presence of irreversible, or slowly reversible, organic changes.

(d) Other factors are involved in the generation of the conventional diagnostic entity, or entities.

The *therapeutic* exclusion diet usually demands the *total* exclusion of offending foods. This is the safest initial course of action. However, it is to be admitted that the matter of *threshold* might be taken into consideration after the patient has improved somewhat. For example, a headache may not be produced by $\frac{1}{2}$ pint ($\frac{1}{4}$ litre) of beer, but the consumption of one pint ($\frac{1}{2}$ litre) may produce a full-blown attack. Where the threshold is readily calculable, these foods may be reintroduced at a sub-threshold level. However, where the threshold level is difficult to assess, it is better to follow the course of total exclusion with regard to the offending substance.

It is also to be borne in mind that the patient may change in his reaction to foods. Particularly in children, one allergy may be lost, and another gained. Alternatively, none may be lost, and others gained. After all, the therapeutic exclusion diet does nothing to remove the *fundamental disease* of origin, be it cellular or genetic.

As I have said previously, the identification and exclusion of allergenic foods is a desirable preparation for the introduction of homoeopathic medicinal remedies. The reduction of toxicity favours the action of these remedies. Homoeopathic remedies are capable of treating the fundamental disease which causes the allergic response. Since there is always a risk that the patient's reaction to foods might change, albeit a slow process, it is of prime importance that we introduce homoeopathic remedies at the earliest possible opportunity. Indeed, this should be done as soon as we have completed our initial trials of a therapeutic exclusion diet. This is generally one or two months after our commencement of this regime.

A final observation. As with hypoglycaemia, there is a direct relationship, in some cases, between food allergy threshold and psychological stress. This is generally more common in adults than children. This is why a method such as hypnosis occasionally reduces or eliminates allergic response.

36.

Dietetic Supplements

Our final major topic with regard to nutritional therapy concerns the use of supplements. In this regard, we shall confine ourselves to the most commonly useful aspects.

Firstly, let us consider the reasons why we might like to use nutritional supplements:

1. The dietetic intake is poor. Obviously it would be better to rectify the matter by placing the patient on the sensible basic diet, and ensuring that adequate quantities of food are consumed. However, there are circumstances where this is not feasible, at least initially:

(a) Socio-economic problems (e.g. alcoholism, poverty).

(b) Partial gastrectomy.

(c) Anorexia.

2. Poor intestinal absorption. This is to be found in:

(a) The elderly.

(b) Pernicious anaemia.

(c) Intestinal hurry, from whatever cause.

3. Increased nutritional demands. These are to be found in:

(a) Pregnancy.

(b) Psychological stress and hypoglycaemia.

(c) Cardiovascular disease.

(d) Endocrine hyperfunction in general.

(e) Acute diseases, or acute exacerbations of chronic disease.

(f) The healing phase of any chronic disease.

(g) Rapid growth phases of childhood.

(h) Pre-menstrual syndrome.

(i) Toxic accumulation (exogenous or endogenous).

4. Inadequate blood supply to tissues, as found in:

(a) Cardiovascular disease.

(b) Sclerotic chronic disease (e.g. osteo-arthritis, fibrosis).

5. Inadequate utilization of nutrients by the cell, as found in:

(a) Chronic disease with severe cellular dysfunction or intracellular disorganization (many advanced chronic diseases, cancer).

(b) Psychoses (e.g. schizophrenia).

(c) Toxic accumulation (exogenous or endogenous).

(d) Endocrine hypofunction in general.

Nutritional supplements include vitamins and minerals. Those that present themselves in the natural state are generally preferable to the synthetic varieties. Those commonly used in homoeopathic practice are:

1. Brewer's yeast and kelp. Often used conjointly to provide a good source of vitamins (especially Vitamin B group) and minerals, including the trace elements. Zinc deficiency is fairly common in young people, and betrays itself by the appearance of white spots on the nails. Brewer's yeast provides a good supply of this mineral. The average dosage of each supplement is ii tabs. bd. For children, the tablets may be crushed. These supplements should be prescribed routinely in pregnancy and lactation. They are often required in the elderly, patients with a sluggish metabolism, and those experiencing excessive psychological stress.

2. Vitamin B^6 (pyridoxine). Demand for this vitamin rises in women on the contraceptive pill, many cases of pre-menstrual syndrome, anxiety states in either sex, and hypoglycaemia. The average adult dose is 50mg bd. Occasionally patients feel unwell on this dosage, but many of these can tolerate, and derive benefit from 10-20mg daily.

3. Cod-liver oil. This is best supplied as capsules, and contains Vitamin A and Vitamin D. Since these vitamins are toxic in high dosage, the patient is advised not to exceed that recommended by the manufacturer. Its particular success is in the treatment of some cases of osteo-arthritis.

4. Vitamin E and lecithin. Both these substances have a protective action on the cardiovascular system, and may, in some instances, even encourage repair. They are often given conjointly, and are used in the therapy of cardiac disorders, arterial disorders, hypertension, and varicose veins. The initial dose of Vitamin E is 100 mg/IU bd. This may be raised in the second month of therapy to 200mg/IU bd, and, in the third month, to 300mg/IU bd. It is seldom necessary to exceed a daily dosage of 600mg/IU. The average dose of lecithin is i capsule bd. Vitamin E is also useful in reducing fibrosis, and scar tissue. Direct application of the contents of a Vitamin E capsule to either burns, or the thin skin that threatens varicose ulceration, encourages healing. Since the content of Vitamin E capsules is oily, when given orally, they should be taken after meals to prevent bloating.

5. Vitamin C. This is the great detoxifying vitamin. It is usefully prescribed during acute infectious disease, allergic reactions (e.g. hay fever, drug rash), and in some cases of cancer. For adults, dosages of up to 10g daily (given in divided doses) may be given for a few days. For maintenance in adults, daily dosages of 1-4g are permissible. Mild cases of hay-fever are sometimes dramatically relieved by this regime.

6. Garlic. Whether this should be regarded as a nutritional supplement or as a natural antibiotic, I am not certain. Nevertheless, it is of great service in the prevention and treatment of the common cold, influenza, and secondary bacterial infection arising therefrom. It may be supplied as garlic tablets, garlic and parsley capsules, or odourless garlic tablets. The preventative dose is usually i tab./caps. daily, the therapeutic dose i tab./caps. bd. Since it is a substance of minimal toxicity, there is little point in worrying about reducing the dose for children. Generally it is wise to swallow garlic preparations with cold water, to reduce odour, which may be offensive to others. Children can generally be induced to nibble garlic tablets. We have previously remarked how garlic can be given transcutaneously. Another substance of peculiar antibiotic property is barley. Given as barley-water or barley-soup, it is useful in the treatment of cystitis.

7. Alfalfa. Not only does this plant have a healing effect on the stomach, it is also of service in the treatment of some cases of arthritis. It is most conveniently supplied in the form of compressed tablets, in a dosage of ii bd or tid.

8. Herbal teas. These may be used in conjunction with other therapies for their mild supportive action. They include:

(a) Peppermint or cardamom in gastric or biliary disorders.
(b) Chamomile for its calming action on the mind.
(c) Skullcap in epilepsy.
(d) Dandelion in mild cases of oedema.

37.

Constitutional and
Pathological Prescribing

Having now completed our discussions on nutrition, we must pass to the application of medicinal remedies to the treatment of chronic disease. For newcomers to homoeopathy, it is generally wise to complete your nutritional adjustments before proceeding to apply remedies. As more expertise is gained, it is often permissible to run nutritional modification and medicinal prescribing conjointly, for this often reduces the treatment time.

Let us first examine our objectives with regard to the therapy of chronic disease:

1. To alleviate the suffering of the patient:
(a) By the reduction of pain or discomfort.
(b) By increasing mobility.
(c) By reducing mental anguish.
(d) By increasing general energy level.
2. To subdue or eliminate fundamental disease.
3. To correct modifying factors where possible.
4. To arrest the disease thereby.
5. To reverse anatomical and physiological change where possible.
6. All these to be done without harm to the patient.

It is a useful exercise for the physician to contemplate the extent to which these ideals are fulfilled by the use of allopathic drugs.

In allopathy, the attention of the physician is largely directed to the alleviation of suffering of the patient. Drugs are applied which have the ability to diminish the force of particular pathological processes. These pathological processes are the prime target for the action of drugs. They are, however, mere end-products of fundamental disease, and little or no attention is paid to the latter.

Whereas it would seem laudable for the physician to relieve immediate suffering by the use of allopathic drugs, it does incur certain serious disadvantages for the patient:

1. The fundamental disease is neither subdued nor eradicated, and thus the patient cannot be 'cured'.

2. Pathological process contains two elements: destruction and healing. Allopathic drugs generally oppose *both* elements. Hence, the alleviation of suffering is accompanied by the *suppression* of healing.

3. The suppression of the healing potential of the body is not without consequence, for it is the ability of the body to heal itself which opposes the action of the fundamental disease. Once healing has been suppressed by drugs, the latter is at liberty to act with even greater vigour. Having been denied expression in one direction, the volcano of fundamental disease will seek a vent in other areas. Hence, the suppression of minor pathology may lead to the development of more serious disease. The vigorous suppression of eczema with steroid creams may induce the onset of asthma. A disease with a large cutaneous expression and mild internal disturbance becomes reversed in its polarity, or *internalized,* as we say.

4. Most drugs are directly toxic. Commonly reported side-effects are generally due to direct toxicity. Individualized and rare side-effects of drugs are more likely due to suppression, rather than direct toxicity, and are a consequence of the fundamental disease seeking different modes of expression.

Chronic disease may be conceptualized as a prolonged battle between the activities of the fundamental disease and the healing processes of the body. Our idea in homoeopathy is to attack the fundamental disease, whilst promoting the healing power of the body itself. We must induce healing from within, so to speak.

Having made the allegation that allopathic drugs are suppressive, can the same be said of homoeopathic remedies? With regard to the applications of *constitutional remedies,* those that attack fundamental disease, this is obviously not so; for they treat disease at its very roots. However, it is also possible to apply *superficial* remedies in the treatment of chronic disease. These are also termed *pathological remedies,* for they seem to have a beneficial action on certain types of pathology, but little direct action on fundamental disease. The use of *Rhus tox.* in the treatment of arthritis is an example.

Now, these pathological remedies can do much to alleviate the suffering of the patient, and, by our own confession, have little direct effect on fundamental disease. They would seem, therefore, to be akin to drugs in these respects. Are they, therefore, to be considered as suppressive in action? The answer is a definite 'No'! You will recall that there are two elements in pathological process: destruction and healing. Homoeopathic remedies work by encouraging the healing component, thus opposing the destructive element. In this way, they are quite different from drugs in their action, and are not to be classified as suppressive.

Thus, pathological remedies, though mainly peripheral in action, maintain and fortify the body's opposition to the fundamental disease. Under such circumstances it will not be induced by our therapeutic measures to break forth elsewhere in the system. Moreover, where the fundamental disease is limited in its mode of expression to one particular pathology, it may be subdued by the action of the simple pathological remedy alone, without the need to apply deep-acting constitutional remedies. However, more often than not, the physician is confronted with cases of much greater pathological complexity, and the patient cannot be 'cured' without the use of constitutional remedies.

You are now aware that remedies may exert their action peripherally (pathological remedies), or centrally (constitutional remedies). Since we have a choice in the matter, how do we decide what to do, and when?

Because of its relevance to the matter, we must initially consider the mode of action of remedies at the physiological level. In simplified terms, they act in two ways, often simultaneously:

(a) They enhance the reactivity of the body to endogenous and exogenous toxins (micro-organisms may be included in the exogenous group). At the bio-chemical level, endogenous toxins are important in the development of chronic disease, and were there no attempt to limit their destructive capabilities, the patient would rapidly expire. An attack of acute gout, albeit a painful experience, at least limits the degree of tissue destruction that would occur if the action of the urate crystals went unopposed.

(b) They promote the elimination of endogenous and exogenous toxins from the body (via gut, kidney, skin, etc).

Should the remedy act largely by enhancing reactivity, then a major *healing crisis* will be experienced. This is an *apparent* worsening of the patient's condition following the administration of the remedy. Thus, increased swelling and pain may be experienced *temporarily* in a case of chronic inflammatory arthritis. Following the crisis, the patient enters an improvement or *healing phase*.

Constitutional remedies are particularly prone to induce healing crisis. Their action on the fundamental disease induces secondary peripheral reactivity. This is largely manifest as apparent exacerbation of the prime pathology, but may also show itself in other areas. These are generally sites of minor pathological expression of the fundamental disease. Moreover, in many cases, these minor outlets of disease are the vestiges of previous major pathological expression, and this is readily deduced from the past history of the patient. Healing crisis may, therefore, be accompanied by the temporary restoration of old symptoms. Since a great deal of energy is required to fire the crisis, the *general energy* pool is sapped. Thus, it is not uncommon for the patient to feel fatigued.

Healing crisis generally occurs 10-14 days after the commencement of constitutional remedial therapy, and often persists for a week or two. In some cases, however, it may begin within an hour or two of giving the first dose of remedy. Alternatively, it may be delayed for a month or more.

Healing crisis following the use of constitutional remedies is very common, but is not necessarily seen in every case. The likelihood of crisis is increased by:

(a) Accurate matching of the remedy to the case.
(b) The use of high potencies (12c and above).
(c) Frequent dose repetition.

The likelihood of crisis is reduced by:

(a) Inaccurate matching of the remedy to the case.
(b) The use of low potencies (6c).
(c) Infrequent dose repetition.

Healing crisis, though essentially the product of the deep-acting constitutional remedies, is occasionally seen in treatment with the superficial pathological remedies. This fact has already been mentioned in connection with the treatment of acute disease. The reaction experienced by the patient, however, is seldom as violent.

Healing crisis is seldom seen in the use of pathological remedies, since their dominant action is to promote the excretion of toxins from the body. This usually occurs through the liver into the biliary tract, through the kidneys, and directly into the gut. At the worst, only minor symptoms are generally produced, such as mild and transient diarrhoea. Thus, healing crisis is uncommon in the treatment of acute disease, since we are largely involved with pathological prescribing.

However, as with everything, it is not all black and white. Constitutional remedies do have some eliminative properties, and pathological remedies do have some ability to promote reactivity. With regard to pathological remedies, this latter property is relatively weak, and is seldom overtly manifest. However, it is sometimes unmasked after the use of prolonged dose repetition.

Let us now examine the relevance of these statements to the question: 'Constitutional, or pathological remedies, which to apply?' Consider the following points:

1. Constitutional therapy is generally the most appropriate to apply initially, for it gets at the roots of the disease.

2. However, constitutional remedies often induce healing crisis. This entails:

(a) Exaggeration of symptoms and signs.

(b) Extra demands placed on the vital organs (heart, endocrine glands, kidneys, etc.).

(c) Sapping of general energy.

(d) Toxic accumulation.

3. In most cases, this crisis is not only harmless, but positively beneficial, for it speeds the patient towards the goal of cure. However, in some cases, it would be undesirable to induce a profound crisis and these may be deduced from points 2a, 2b, 2c and 2d:

(a) Where the patient is already in a state of great pain or discomfort (e.g. rheumatoid arthritis), and it would be inadvisable to worsen the misery, even temporarily.

(b) Where the site of the prime pathology renders it potentially hazardous to life (e.g. very severe cases of asthma).

(c) Where the vital organs, such as the heart, are grossly diseased, and could not take the strain of crisis.

(d) Where the general energy level of the patient is extremely low as a result of prolonged generalized chronic disease, or prolonged nutritional deficiency.

(e) Conditions (c) and (d), given above, prevail in the elderly, and constitutional remedies are to be applied only with great caution and experience.

(f) In pregnancy and lactation.

(g) In children under six months of age, for fear of disturbing their intake of food. Constitutional remedies may be used here, but great caution must be observed in their application.

4. In diseases of many years duration, constitutional prescribing is *sometimes* without effect. The disease is 'burnt out', so to speak. The fundamental disease is absent or dormant. The patient, though presenting with anatomical and physiological disturbance, often to a great degree, shows little or no sign of disease progression. The case is virtually static. Because the fun-

damental disease has ceased to act, the application of constitutional remedies is ineffective and unwarranted. Should this be the state of affairs in an elderly patient, no harm, yet no good, will come of constitutional prescribing.

5. The prescription of pathological remedies is indicated in the following situations:

(a) Where the generation of a major healing crisis might be undesirable (see 3 a-g). Healing crisis is rare with the use of pathological remedies. When it does occur, it is of a minor nature, and rapidly abates when the remedy is discontinued. Should, however, the physiological state of the patient at risk change for the better, then the introduction of constitutional treatment subsequently is desirable. In this sense, pathological prescribing may be a preparation for the application of constitutional therapy at a later date.

(b) In 'burnt out' cases (see 4).

(c) After constitutional therapy, to finish the case. Constitutional therapy, by virtue of its action on fundamental disease, often induces the case to become 'burnt out'. After many months, it becomes apparent that no further improvement with constitutional therapy is likely. The case plateaus out, so to speak. The residual organic and physiological changes require the action of the peripherally acting pathological remedies. In other cases, the selected constitutional therapy has been only partially effective in dealing with the fundamental disease. This may be due to difficulties in correct remedy selection or failure to identify and remove modifying factors. The physician is then committed to the utilization of pathological remedies.

(d) In conjunction with constitutional therapy, in order to reinforce the action of the latter at the periphery. This is a tricky technique for the newcomer to homoeopathy to master, for it requires a good knowledge of the compatibility and complementary relationships of remedies. The direct peripheral action of the pathological remedy complements the secondary peripheral action of the constitutional remedy. You will recall that these two types of remedies are of opposite polarity with respect to the promotion of reactivity and the promotion of detoxification. In some texts, the latter facility is termed 'drainage', and this is the forte of the pathological remedy. The pathological remedy fortifies the weaker detoxification property of the constitutional remedy.

(e) Where there has been great difficulty in finding a constitutional remedy. The physician is then compelled to resort to the use of pathological remedies.

Since pathological prescribing has little or no effect on fundamental disease, it is seldom curative in its own right. Nevertheless, used by itself, it can bring the relief of much suffering, though the patient is generally committed to an indefinite course of therapy.

Constitutional prescribing must obviously be considered as a superior method with regard to the goal of cure, but is not without limitations, and these have been specified. In simple cases, and these are often diseases of childhood, the application of a single well-chosen constitutional remedy cures. More frequently, especially in adults, where the disease is more complex, several different constitutional and pathological remedies are required to complete the case.

Additionally, it must be stated that pathological remedies often act with greater vigour after the application of well-chosen constitutional remedies.

Whereas exceptions to this rule have been stated, it is generally desirable to initiate the case with constitutional prescribing, and this matter we shall now discuss in some detail.

38.
General Constitutional
Prescribing

Constitutional remedies attack fundamental disease, and are, therefore, also termed *deep-acting*. Though there is some overlap of action, for the purposes of discussion, they may be divided into two main types:
1. General constitutional remedies.
2. Antimiasmatic remedies.

As we have noted, a *miasm* is the physiological (or anatomophysiological) aftermath of an infectious illness, and remedies that correct the fundamental disease therein may be termed *antimiasmatic*. Since the application of these remedies warrants special consideration, we shall, for the moment restrict ourselves to the matter of *general constitutional remedies*.

You will recall that remedies for the treatment of acute disease are selected largely on the individualized characteristics of the acute disturbance, little regard being paid to the general make-up of the person. The same largely applies to the prescription of pathological remedies in chronic disease, where the minutiae of the presenting complaint determine the choice of remedy.

In contradistinction, the general characteristics of the patient, including his past history, are of prime importance in the selection of a constitutional remedy, the minutiae of the presenting complaint being relegated to a position of secondary importance.

These most important general characteristics are termed the *generals* of the case, as opposed to details of the presenting complaint, which are termed the *particulars*. At first sight, it may seem illogical to take the generals in preference to the particulars in order to determine a prescription. But our object in constitutional therapy is to treat the 'ground' in which the presenting disease grows, rather than the tree itself. In that way, we influence its growth at the roots, and, indeed, of any other pathological tree that might be growing in the same soil. In contrast, pathological prescribing largely treats the tree directly.

The *generals,* given in descending order of importance with regard to remedy selection, may be classified thus:

(a) The *mentals*.
(b) General modalities.
(c) Desires and aversions.
(d) Pathological predispositions.
(e) Anatomical structure.

The *mentals* constitute the general psychological make-up of the patient. These include such things as: emotional lability, dislike of consolation, depressive tendencies, emotional reactions to music, fear, demanding love, cruelty, philosophical nature, self-interest, perfectionism, excessive loquacity, claustrophobia, sexual disinclination, etc.

The mentals are generally held to be of the highest significance with regard to constitutional remedial selection, but this is so only if they are *well-defined*. In homoeopathy, constitutional types are defined by their corresponding remedies. *Pulsatilla* types are passive, with emotional (and physical) liability. *Natrum muriaticum* types are depressive, with a dislike of consolation. *Arsenicum album* types are depressive, with perfectionistic behaviour, and thus are always well-dressed; even their casual attire is meticulously chosen.

Depending upon the mentals, some remedies are better indicated in one sex rather than the other. Thus, *Pulsatilla* is more commonly prescribed in women than in men, partially because passivity, emotional liability, and tearfulness are features more commonly seen in them. However, there are also many men of *Pulsatilla* type, but, unlike the women, some may attempt to cover up their emotional status in order to preserve male ego. You may have to drag it out of them, so to speak.

Occupation is always an important question with regard to the mentals. Its nature may assist us in determining the character of the patient, provided, of course, that he has been able to select a job suited to his own mental requirements. *Sulphur* types, who are generally of a philosophical nature, tend to choose work with a strong theoretical element (e.g. lecturing). *Phosphorus* types show a definite affinity for other people, and seek work accordingly (e.g. personnel work, nursing). *Nux vomica* types seek the hectic world of commerce.

Where force of circumstances has driven the patient into a particular occupation, the latter will not assist us in determining his basic character. Here, we must question the patient about his out-of-work interests. Hence, a banker may be an avid reader of history in his spare time. He became a banker because his father was one. He may, thus, be better suited to *Sulphur* rather than *Nux vomica* from the constitutional aspect.

This brings us to another matter of some importance. This is the changeability of constitution within the individual as determined by the mentals. In childhood, constitutional changes, at both physical and mental levels, are common. The fat and docile *Calcarea carbonica* infant, may change into the tall, slim, and outward-going Phosphoric child. After the teens, however, the mentals tend to stabilize into a well-observed pattern.

With regard to adult patients, therefore, it is these stable patterns of mental status that we must determine with regard to constitutional prescribing. We must ignore little nuances of thought and behaviour. To take a recent episode of depression into consideration, in a patient who is fundamentally happy by nature, may be good from the point of view of pathological prescription, but is of little use in constitutional prescribing.

In contrast, short term changes of mental status (a few months or more), preceding or in conjunction with the presenting complaint, must be considered as relevant to the selection of a constitutional remedy *in childhood* and in many teenage cases. However, in some circumstances, the influence of the environment is sufficiently strong and prolonged to produce considerable change of the mentals in adult life. A new stable pattern emerges. Hence, our philosophical Sulphuric banker, after many years in an inappropriate occupation, may become a neurotic, aggressive businessman in consequence, with little time for reading. His type will have changed from *Sulphur* towards *Nux vomica*.

Should it be considered that the presenting complaint might well have arisen in association with the new stable set of mentals, then *Nux vomica* is more likely the constitutional remedy. If, however, the presenting complaint was present before the onset of the new set of mentals, then the previous mentals, those that correspond to *Sulphur,* should be considered as more relevant.

In some of these cases, the patient presents with a mixture of complaints preceding the change of character, and those associated with the latter. In such circumstances, we are obliged to apply two constitutional remedies in sequence. The first constitutional remedy is generally that which corresponds to the present mental status (*Nux vomica*), and the one applied later is that which corresponds to the previous mental status (*Sulphur*).

It is a fact of life that for every mental disturbance, there is a physical manifestation, and *vice versa*. Whenever there is a definite change of what might be termed *mental constitution,* there is a definite change of *physical constitution.* A constitutional remedy must match both aspects of the case. Whilst the mental aspects are of prime importance, they must be considered together with the physical for the constitutional prescription to be effective. Homoeopathy not only recognizes the integral nature of mind and body, it utilizes this notion to determine its remedies.

In some texts, the mentals are erroneously described as *mental symptoms.* Some, it is true, are pathological, such as chronic depression, and may be regarded as *symptoms.* Others, however, such as a philosophical nature, could hardly be considered as symptoms of disease. Whilst some mentals are symptomatic, and therefore alterable, others are fixed, and unalterable. We may cure chronic depression, but we are unlikely to remove a philosophical predisposition. Should we thus ignore the fixed and unalterable mentals when we come to seek a constitutional remedy? It is a matter of experience that we should not. For the affinity of remedies to the patient is as much determined by the fixed as the alterable mentals. Similarly, with regard to physical constitution, there are both fixed and modifiable aspects. We cannot change the colour of the eyes, but we are able to correct a mild squint. The homoeopath is not a Baron Frankenstein.

Next in importance are the *general modalities.* These are those things or circumstances that make the patient feel generally better or worse. These include: changes in environment (snow, damp, stuffy atmospheres, etc.), types of food (e.g. fat), and times of the day or year (seasonal changes). *Pulsatilla* types react badly to stuffy atmospheres, and are improved by the open air. *Lycopodium* types are often at their worst between 4 p.m. and 8 p.m.

Desires and aversions are often closely related to the general modalities, since we tend to desire that which makes us feel better, and avoid that which makes us worse. They may also be regarded as part of the mentals. *Pulsatilla* types often react badly to fat, and generally have a loathing of it. However, some *Pulsatilla* types react badly to fats, but still have a desire to eat them, perhaps because they were brought up on them. *Calcarea carbonica* children have a great desire to eat indigestible things, such as coal and pencils. *Arsenicum album* types are made worse by cold, and thus have an aversion to it.

Pathological predisposition is revealed by taking a careful case history back to birth. *Phosphorus* types are prone to recurrent attacks of bronchitis. *Sulphur* types are prone to recurrent boils, and recurrent skin complaints in general. *Pulsatilla* types are prone to varicose veins. Where the predisposition still exists, it is of great significance in constitutional prescribing. Where the predisposition existed in the past, but has apparently disappeared, it still must be considered as relevant to prescribing, for it may have been a manifestation of the same fundamental disease that still acts, and causes the presenting complaint.

Anatomical structure also has its relevance. The *Calcarea carbonica* type tends to be short and fat, with stubby fingers, whilst the *Phosphorus* type tends to be tall and thin, with slender hands. The *Lycopodium* type is wizened in appearance, and seems older than his years.

Having assessed these generals, we must define any *peculiar* or *characteristic* symptoms of the patient. These are symptoms of unusual nature that give the case great individuality. They may be found as part of the generals or the particulars. 'Burning pain relieved by heat' is such a peculiar symptom, and suggests the remedy *Arsenicum album*. Should the remainder of the case tally with the properties of the latter, then it would be considered to be the correct constitutional remedy. Peculiar symptoms serve to accelerate our method of remedy selection, by pointing us to one or two particular remedies. Whereas we should never prescribe on the basis of the peculiar symptom alone, it is a clinical fact that, more often than not, the implicated remedy will match the remainder of the case.

A knowledge of the peculiar symptoms can only come by careful study of *materia medica,* and the use of *repertories*. Regrettably, many cases lack anything that could be called a peculiar symptom, and they may also lack any well-defined mentals. Should this be so, we must rely on careful observation of general modalities, desires and aversions, pathological predispositions, and anatomical structure, in order to select a remedy.

Whilst the *particulars* of the case are relegated to a minor position in constitutional remedy selection, they are, however, not without use. We have already noted that peculiar symptoms are of great importance, and may be found amongst the particulars. Additionally, where a modality of the presenting complaint corresponds to a general modality, this serves to reinforce the importance of the modality in selecting the constitutional remedy. A patient, since childhood, has always felt ill during thundery weather. Her arthritis, present for two years, is always more painful during thundery weather. The modality 'worse for thundery weather' should, therefore, be covered by the selected deep-acting remedy, perhaps *Phosphorus*. Similarly, where the presenting complaint is part of a general pathological predisposition, this too serves to emphasize the importance of the latter in remedy selection.

Having taken the observable *totality* of the case, we must select the most significant and well-defined facts. These, in turn, must be matched against the known properties of remedies as defined in the *materia medica*. We are assisted in this matter by the use of *repertories,* a matter which has been previously outlined. But these cannot act as substitutes for the *materia medica* itself.

We must match the *well-defined aspects of the case* against the *well-defined properties of remedies*.

The first thing to be said in this respect, is that the *materia medica* contains details of numerous remedies totally unsuited to our task. Through insufficient usage, their properties are not well-defined at all, and we are merely reading the results of a few clinical studies, or accidental provings. Others have a well-documented pathological application, but a poorly confirmed set of constitutional indications. It is to be realized that, whereas the Law of Similars is the very foundation of homoeopathy, only *clinical usage* in many cases over a prolonged period (many years), can, and must demonstrate the relevance of our *provings* to the treatment of our patients.

The Law of Similars *indicates* the probable application of a remedy. Clinical usage *confirms* it. Clinical usage is, by the way, not the same as *clinical trial* in the allopathic sense. Recently, much doubt has been cast upon the scientific validity of allopathic drug trials, which certainly did nothing to forewarn the victims of *benoxaprofen!* Clinical usage is more reliable and thorough a method. It results in the accumulation of knowledge derived from thousands of remedial prescriptions issued over a large number of years; fifty to a hundred, or more, in many cases.

The newcomer to homoeopathy is, therefore, strongly advised to restrict his constitutional prescribing to the *major* remedies of the *materia medica*. The identity of these, and their indications are discussed in the next dialogue. These remedies are well-tried and tested.

The next point of issue is our ability to match *all* the well-defined aspects of our case against those of a major remedy. In many cases, this is not possible, and we must compromise. We must settle for a match of the majority of those aspects of the case against a particular remedy, which effectively becomes the constitutional remedy. In this respect, correlation between case and remedy is usually better achieved in the child, who is often less complex than the adult.

Fortunately, even subtotal matching is with good clinical effect. The results of the application of the first remedy (the first constitutional *similimum*) often sufficiently simplify the case, so that the selection of further *similima* is not too difficult a task. In the child, the subtotally matched remedy may bring the case to a beneficial conclusion by its own action alone.

You will have observed that some of the remedies that have been mentioned in connection with constitutional treatment have also been discussed with regard to acute disease therapy (e.g. *Pulsatilla*). Their constitutional activity is only revealed when their properties match the generals of the case at hand. Their pathological activity is only revealed when they match the particulars of the case at hand.

The term *susceptible typology* refers to those aspects of anatomical conformation, overt temperament, and pathology, that would lead you, in the very earliest stages of examination and history-taking, to the consideration of a particular constitutional remedy. Thus, a weepy young lady, with erythrocyanosis, and an appearance rather younger than her years, might suggest the remedy *Pulsatilla*. These points may be observed often within minutes of the patient entering the consulting room. As you become more experienced, and your knowledge of *materia medica* increases, so you will be able to develop this facility. Obviously, an appreciation of susceptible typology greatly simplifies the selection of a constitutional remedy. In many cases, a few pertinent questions will satisfy the practitioner that his initial choice was a correct one.

39.

Major General
Constitutional Remedies

In actual clinical practice, the selection of the appropriate general constitutional *similimum* is frequently made with regard to:

(a) Susceptible typology.

(b) Peculiar (characteristic) symptoms.

Since peculiar (characteristic) symptoms lead one to consider a restricted number of remedies, of which they are characteristic, they are also termed *keynote* symptoms. They are not, however, always true symptoms of disease, and may be fixed aspects of the person. Moreover, keynotes may be found within the category of susceptible typology. The fastidiousness of attire, characteristic of the *Arsenicum album* type, is a keynote to be extracted from the susceptible typology; and, whilst it cannot be regarded as a symptom of disease, unless inconsistent with the former character of the patient, it may well suggest a susceptibility to the action of *Arsenicum album*.

In general, it is inadvisable to rely solely upon a particular keynote in order to issue a prescription. In contrast, prescribing based upon a synthesis of keynote and typology often yields favourable results. Remember that susceptible typology does include at least a superficial appraisal of temperament (the mentals). It is not simply a matter of morphology (anatomical structure), and pathological predisposition.

This simplified approach to general constitutional prescribing is both a manageable tool for the tyro, and a reasonably successful one in actual practice. It is, therefore, to be encouraged in preference to the often vain attempts to squeeze the totality of the case into the Procrustean bed of a single remedy. For, in order to achieve this 'quart into a pint pot', it is frequently necessary to match the minor symptomatology of the patient with the major characteristics of the remedy, and vice versa. This is totally unrealistic, since a natural corollary of the Law of Similars must be to match *emphasis* of the case at hand with *emphasis* of properties of the remedy, as delineated within the *materia medica*. Hence, all initial studies of the latter made by the physician should be orientated towards the major properties of remedies, and study of the 'small print' left in abeyance. In the brief accounts that follow, I will endeavour to outline only a few major properties of each general constitutional remedy, this being consistent with the former sentiments.

This list is intended to be neither complete with regard to the number of possible general constitutional remedies, nor with regard to the properties of each. It will, however, serve as a base for the newcomer, and an introduction to the further study of the *materia medica*:

1. ARSENICUM ALBUM

(a) Meticulous, orderly, perfectionistic, agitated, despairing, 'snazzily' dressed.

(b) Pale and thin, with dry and scaly skin.

(c) Chilly (modality: worse for cold).

(d) Great weakness, often out of all proportion to presenting complaint.

(e) Worse in general, or with regard to presenting complaint, between midnight and 3 a.m.

(f) Burning sensations, paradoxically *better* for heat.

(g) Periodicity of complaints marked (e.g. tend to recur every 3 days).

(h) Alternation of cutaneous and internal manifestations (they occur independently, rather than concurrently).

(g) Pathological predispositions: psoriasis, dandruff, thin anterior nasal discharge (often allergic), oedema, history of pityriasis rosea.

2. CALCAREA CARBONICA.

(a) Short, fat individuals with stubby fingers; fat, flabby children.

(b) Easily discouraged and timid.

(c) Chilly.

(d) Sweat profuse from scalp (they soak their pillows at night).

(e) Cold, damp feet.

(f) Intense desire for eggs, and (in children) indigestible substances: chalk, pencils, coal, etc.

(g) Intense desire or aversion to milk, which disagrees.

(h) Aversion to meat. Desire for sweets.

(i) Aggravation by full moon.

(j) Pathological predispositions: gastro-intestinal upsets, cervical lymphadenopathy, polypi, urinary and biliary lithiasis, hypertension, retarded eruption of teeth.

3. CALCAREA PHOSPHORICA

(a) Tall and thin; elegant morphology.

(b) Sensitive, timid, wishes to be left alone.

(c) Intelligent, but easily tired by intellectual work.

(d) 'Growing pains' at ends of long bones, and in back.

(e) Precocious puberty.

(f) Enlarged, pale tonsils.

(g) Precocious puberty in females.

(h) Chilly.

(i) Pathological predispositions: menorrhagia of puberty, juvenile acne, recurrent tonsillitis, chronic cervical lymphadenopathy.

4. GELSEMIUM.

(a) Emotional, jumpy, full of fears, depressive, prone to trepidation (anxiety of anticipation), which may cause diarrhoea.

(b) General muscular weakness.

(c) Diplopia.

(d) Tremor

(e) Vertigo, band-like feeling around head, severe occipital headache, orbital neuralgia.

(f) Pathological predispositions, migraine, paralysis.

5. GRAPHITES

(a) Fat, chilly, dyspeptic, constipated, melancholic.

(b) Dry, thick hair, and thick nails, which break easily.

(c) Delayed periods, and hoarseness of voice during periods.

(d) Absence of sweating.

(e) Moist cutaneous vesicular eruptions; discharge like honey; pruritis ameliorated by cold applications.

(f) Pathological predispositions: eczema (moist), chronic constipation, haemorrhoids with painful fissure, periungual verrucae, keloids, erection with loss of ability to ejaculate.

6. IGNATIA

(a) Rapid alternation of mental state, emotionally hypersensitive, hysterical.

(b) Ill-effects of prolonged grief.

(c) Globus hystericus.

(d) Paradoxical and labile symptoms: globus hystericus worse for liquids rather than solids, hunger not ameliorated by eating, etc.

(e) Disorders tend to be functional, rather than organic.

7. LACHESIS

(a) Fat and plethoric, with great loquacity.

(b) Marked menopausal symptoms.

(c) Hot flushes.

(d) Choking sensations.

(e) Sleeps into aggravation: awakes at night choking.

(f) Cannot bear tight clothing.

(g) Ailments left sided, or travel from left to right (e.g. hip pain).

(h) Aversion to heat.

(i) Pre-menstrual symptoms relieved by the flow.

(j) Pathological predispositions: asthma, varicose ulcers, black erysipelas, tonsillitis (left moving to right), hypertension, spontaneous ecchymoses.

8. LYCOPODIUM

(a) Wizened appearance, making patient seem older than years; narrow thorax with large abdomen.

(b) Melancholic, afraid to be alone.

(c) Flatulence, with *lower* abdominal distension.

(d) Complaints mainly right-sided.

(e) Worse between 4 p.m. and 8 p.m.

(f) Urinary lithiasis, with red grit in urine.

(g) Hair prematurely grey.

(h) Foul sweat.

(i) Burning sensation between shoulder blades.

(j) One foot hot, the other cold.

(k) Cannot tolerate own children.

(l) Impotence, dryness of vagina.

(m) Intellectually keen, physically weak.

(n) Pathological predispositions: urinary and biliary lithiasis, duodenal ulcer, anorexia of children, atherosclerotic hypertension, hyperuricaemia, psoriasis, recurrent urticaria, migraine.

9. MERCURIUS SOLUBILIS

(a) May be timid and morose, or psychopathically destructive (delinquent).

(b) Foul breath and excessive salivation.

(c) Skin constantly moist.

(d) Worse at night.

(e) Sensitive to both heat and cold ('human thermometer').

(f) Intense thirst for cold drinks.

(g) Continuous hunger.

(h) Sneezes in sunshine.

(i) Pathological predispositions: recurrent tonsillitis, chronic periodontitis, green leucorrhoea.

10. NATRUM MURIATICUM

(a) Thin, despite good appetite.

(b) Depressive, with dislike of consolation, which makes the patient worse.

(c) Chilly, but dislike of heat and stuffy atmospheres.

(d) Blinding headaches, in morning on awakening, after periods, from sunrise to sunset.

(e) Craving for salt.

(f) Worse at the seaside.

(g) Skin of face oily.

(h) Vertical fissure of lower lip.

(i) Great thirst.

(j) Sweats whilst eating.

(k) Numbness and tingling in fingers and legs.

(l) Low backache with desire for firm support.

(m) Geographical tongue.

(n) Pathological predispositions: herpes, eczema, acne vulgaris, depressive illness, recurrent headaches, loss of weight, urticaria, verrucae of palms or creases of fingers.

11. NUX VOMICA

(a) Hypersensitive, nervous, irritable, impatient, dislike of contradiction, chilly.

(b) Ill-effects of executive occupations, or sedentary office jobs.

(c) Prone to over-indulgence in food, alcohol, coffee, tea, spices.

(d) Great somnolence after meals.

(e) Helped by a short nap, if allowed to finish it.

(f) Very prone to gastric disturbance.

(g) Constipated.

(h) Insomnia: awakes at about 4 a.m., thinking about work problems.

(i) Pathological predispositions: peptic ulcer, haemorrhoids, recurrent headaches, including migraine, intermittent arterial hypertension, alcoholism.

12. PHOSPHORUS

(a) Tall, thin, sometimes stooped subjects.

(b) Very communicative, and fix you with their eyes, yet the depths of their personality are difficult to extract. They like to be 'magnetized'.

(c) Great thirst for cold drinks.

(d) Aggravation by thundery weather (it often brings on a headache); relieved after the storm.

(e) Great sensitivity to bright lights and loud noises.

(f) Sensitive, rather than timid; often artistic.

(g) Burning pain between the shoulder blades.

(h) Desire for salt.

(i) Clairvoyance.

(j) Worse for lying on the left side.

(k) At night: short naps and frequent wakings.

(l) Numbness of arms and hands.

(m) Joints suddenly give way.

(n) Wounds bleed easily; bruises easily.

(o) Pathological predispositions: hepatic disease, glaucoma, vertigo, recurrent chest infections, haemorrhagic disorders, tuberculosis, nephritis, inflammatory arthritis.

13. PULSATILLA

(a) Mild, yielding, tearful, passive.

(b) Better for consolation.

(c) Girlish appearance of women.

(d) Erythrocyanosis of extremities.

(e) Love of open air, which improves complaints.

(f) Aversion to stuffy atmospheres, but chilly.

(g) Usually an aversion to fat.

(h) Thirstlessness with all complaints.

(i) Two or three stools daily.

(j) Discharge thick, green or yellow-green, and bland (nasal catarrh, vaginal discharge).

(k) Changeable and delicate, emotionally and physically; easily 'tipped'.

(l) Late periods, irregular periods, or amenorrhoea.

(m) Pathological predispositions: irritable bowel syndrome, urticaria, recurrent headaches, chronic nasal catarrh, recurrent vaginal thrush, inflammatory arthritis, varicose veins, chilblains, depressive illness, acne.

14. SEPIA (Cuttlefish ink).

(a) Thin, even feels chilly in a warm room.

(b) Yellowish saddle across nose.

(c) Crack in middle of lower lip.

(d) Avoids crowds.

(e) Depressive, irritable, easily offended.

(f) Indifferent and aggressive to those close to her (husband, children, etc).

(g) Aversion to sexual matters.

(h) Worse for prolonged sedentary work (e.g. doing the washing), but better for exercise.

(i) Worse during pregnancy, breast-feeding, and before periods.

(j) Worse before a storm.

(k) Ball-like sensation of inner parts (e.g. rectum).

(l) Bearing-down sensation of uterus.

(m) Dyspepsia, with hollow feeling of stomach.

(n) Pathological predispositions: depressive illness, herpes, psoriasis, eczema, falling hair, prolapse of uterus, haemorrhoids, premenstrual syndrome.

15. SILICEA

(a) Sickly children, with large abdomen, prominent forehead, and cervical lymphadenopathy.

(b) Multiple white spots on nails, which split easily.

(c) Intelligent and capable, but doubt of own abilities; timid, with anxiety of anticipation.

(d) Chilly, even during exercise.

(e) Profuse sweat of head.

(f) Cold and sweaty feet, with offensive perspiration.

(g) Tendency to catch repeated colds (deficient immune system).

(h) Measles (or measles immunization) causes severe illness (this is a great clue!).

(i) Straining at stool, which recedes after partial expulsion.

(j) Icy coldness during and before menses.

(k) Constipation always before and during menses.

(l) Worse at new moon.

(m) Tendency to cutaneous suppuration.

(n) Somnambulism.

(o) Pathological predispositions: delayed dentition, disorders of ossification, failure to thrive, rickets, periodic quinsy, recurrent bronchitis, tuberculosis.

16. SULPHUR

(a) Philosophical, very selfish.

(b) Burning sensations: burning in hands and soles at night.

(c) Aggravation from the heat of the bed; may stick feet out of bedclothes.

(d) Ebullitions of heat.

(e) Dislike of water.

(f) Dry and hard hair and skin.

(g) Redness and irritation of orifices (mouth, anus, vulva, etc.).

(h) Sinking feeling in stomach at about 11 a.m.

(i) Ragged or ill-dressed.

(j) Worse for standing in one position.

(k) Tendency to relapse of all conditions.

(l) Prone to persistent or recurrent cutaneous affections (e.g. eczema, boils, carbuncles).

(m) Intense pruritis.

(n) Periodicity of complaints.

(o) Alternation of cutaneous and internal manifestations.

(p) May be dirty (dislike of water).

(q) Discharges offensive.

(r) Painless morning diarrhoea, driving patient out of bed.

(s) Better for dry, warm weather.

(t) Desire for sweet things and alcohol.

(u) Pathological predispositions: alcoholism, eczema, recurrent boils and styes, acne vulgaris, arterial hypertension, atherosclerosis, hyperuricaemia.

40.

The Selection of Potency

Whereas you may not appreciate the overall significance of the details specified until you come to view your cases in the homoeopathic manner, you will have gathered that there is a certain degree of overlap in the fields of action of the various remedies. For example, both *Sulphur* and *Arsenicum album* types show periodicity and alternation; yet one is meticulous, whilst the other is disorderly. This is all well and good, for such is the individuality of Man that there is not a clear-cut distinction between one man and his brother. Moreover, the physician can no more choose his patients than he can his relatives, and few patients will fall into an exact category, wherein all the details match those of a particular remedy, especially bearing in mind the matter of emphasis, hitherto discussed. Our objective must be to match as closely as possible, not necessarily exactly. In this way do we determine the general constitutional remedy; an initial one at least.

It would be logical to progress to a consideration of how we should apply our selected constitutional remedy; and so we shall. However, in order to do so, we must reconsider the matter of *potency*.

In the first part of this text, the statement was made that there exists a direct relationship between potency and magnitude of action. This, however, is an over-simplification, in order to prevent confusion to the initiate. Whilst largely true, it now requires some modification.

Whilst the quantification of therapeutic action requires further investigation, the following guidelines may be stated with regard to the relationship of potencies:

A) 30c is about twice as strong as 6c.

(b) 200c is about twice as strong as 30c.

(c) 10M is about twice as strong as 200c.

(d) Little increase in therapeutic action can be expected with potencies above CM.

(e) 6c is approximately equivalent to 9x in terms of therapeutic action.

However, these facts themselves are also an over simplification of the matter. For a lot depends on the way in which the remedy acts. Whilst remedies acting in a general constitutional manner show progressive increase in therapeutic strength as they rise in potency to CM, the same cannot be said of pathological remedies, those that act on the periphery.

Pathologically applied remedies seem to have a level of potency considerably lower than CM, at which they deliver maximal therapeutic action. This peak level appears to vary from remedy to remedy, but, in general, can be taken to be around 200c to 1M. Up to this peak there is the same progressive increase in therapeutic action as with remedies acting on the general constitution. Beyond the peak, however, the remedy will decline in its efficacy. Hence, *Arnica* 10M is therapeutically weaker than *Arnica* 200, provided, of course, that the remedy is acting only on the periphery, which is usually the case with this particular one.

Antimiasmatic remedies show a similar tendency to peak in action at 200c to 1M. Hence, the remedy *Tuberculinum,* used in the treatment of a tuberculous miasm, is seldom used above 200.

The matter becomes more complex when we come to consider the remedy that is well-matched to *both* the generals and the particulars of the case. Such a general constitutional remedy has additional properties. It has the ability to exert a *direct* peripheral action on the case, and, therefore, to induce detoxification to a significant degree. It acts as its own 'drainer', so to speak. That is to say, if we allow it to do so. For the detoxification effect will diminish beyond the level of 200c to 1M, and prescriptions in excess of 1M will diminish its peripheral powers.

There is also another problem. General constitutional remedies that are particularly well-matched to the generals of the case will often show a fair degree of antimiasmatic effect. The latter will be reduced by prescribing potencies in excess of 1M.

It is sometimes erroneously stated that low potencies cause aggravation, and high potencies do not. Furthermore, others have stated that homoeopathic aggravation (healing crisis) is a rare phenomenon in general. Both these misconceptions stem from a misapprehension of the different ways in which remedies can act. Invariably, the protagonists of these suspect concepts have referred to pathological prescribing experiences, under the guise of constitutional therapy. A remedy that does not attack fundamental disease is not likely to cause aggravation.

Moreover, since these pseudo-constitutional prescriptions are often given in very high potency, in the belief that they are truly constitutional, they are given beyond the peak of maximal therapeutic effect.

Those rare healing crises that do occur with pathological remedies are, of course, more likely to occur in the range 6c to 200c, for a 10M potency of a pathological remedy may be weaker in effect than a 6c. Another contributory factor in the generation of the fear of low potencies is the fact that *crude substance* (unpotentized material) is capable of producing considerable aggravation. This, however, only applies to highly toxic substances, such as Arsenic, and is due to direct chemical poisoning. Such an effect is totally removed in the early stages of serial dilution, by the elimination of original substance. Whilst a 2x potency of toxic material is still capable of direct chemical aggravation, a 6c is not.

Whilst direct chemical aggravation is something to be avoided, healing crisis is not necessarily something to be feared. Whereas it should be avoided in certain cases, as I have described previously, in the majority of cases it is of immense benefit to the patient in the long-term.

41.

Practical Aspects
of General Constitutional Prescribing,
and the Law of Cure

Having selected our general constitutional remedy, and having familiarized ourselves with the matter of potency, we must now determine the way in which we should administer it.

Bearing in mind all that has been said with regard to potency, a safe and effective method is to administer the remedy in 12c potency, twice daily. This is a good all-round system. The patient is generally reviewed in one month, but modifications to the regime may be needed before the month is up, and these can often be carried out over the telephone. Let us discuss the various possible consequences of our first month of treatment, and what actions to take in accordance:

1. Remedy given twice daily for one month, yet neither aggravation nor improvement detectable. In this situation, we have a totally mismatched remedy on our hands. The remedy must be changed. Alternatively, there is a gross nutritional or toxic factor present which we have failed to identify, and which inhibits the action of a correctly selected remedy. Do not use this as an excuse, however, for what is normally poor prescribing. Another possibility is that we have failed to realize that the case is essentially 'burnt out' (fundamental disease inactive).

2. Remedy given twice daily, with initial improvement (this usually occurs within seven days). Here the remedy is working, but the detoxification function has become manifest before the reactive function. This improvement phase is generally followed by a healing crisis, as the reactive function comes into play. However, in some instances, the improvement phase continues for the remainder of the month, with no sign of crisis. Whilst, in rare cases, the crisis may be delayed until the second month, in most instances we must assume that we have prescribed a remedy that acts in the pathological sense, rather than the constitutional. Nevertheless, whatever the cause of our improvement phase, the remedy must be continued throughout it in the twice daily dosage.

3. Remedy given twice daily, and healing crisis occurs (generally at about 7-10 days). As has been stated, it may be

preceded by an initial improvement stage. The remedy is now attacking the fundamental disease. Since we do not wish to over-promote the healing mechanisms of the body, the remedy must be stopped if the patient is considerably distressed by the crisis. This must be done immediately. However, where the crisis is well-tolerated by the patient, it is generally advisable to inform him to continue on the twice daily dosage for the remainder of the month, unless the crisis increases to an uncomfortable level, in which case he should stop taking the remedy.

We are utilizing the patient himself as a gauge of the level of crisis that is acceptable from his point of view and ours. The crisis usually lasts from 2-7 days, after which it abates. In cases of severe crisis, this occurs with discontinuation of the remedy. It also occurs where the remedy is continued through a phase of mild crisis.

By the time the patient is reviewed at one month, he is generally through the crisis, and into an improvement phase. Remember to inform all patients, prior to the commencement of treatment, that they must contact you for advice should healing crisis occur. If you are not available for advice, and they feel that the crisis is severe, they must realize that the safest course of action is to discontinue the remedy. This they will do if you inform them of these matters before the treatment is started.

The patient is now reviewed at the end of the first month. What to do next? If there has been neither aggravation nor improvement, and we are satisfied that there is no significant interference from nutritional or toxic factors, then it is well to stop the original remedy and prescribe a pathological remedy. This is useful where either the selection of a constitutional remedy has been difficult (cases with a lack of well-defined generals), or the case is 'burnt out'. The selection of a remedy based on the particulars is, as a rule, a simpler task. On the other hand, where the patient has entered an improvement phase by the time of consultation, it is best to maintain the *status quo*. That is to say, where the remedy has been discontinued because of potent healing crisis, do not represcribe, and where the patient still takes the remedy (healing crisis has been mild, or remedy acts pathologically), this should be continued as before.

This *status quo* is best maintained as long as the patient continues to improve. The patient should generally be reviewed every month, but must feel free to contact the practitioner by post or telephone, should he have any problems between visits. Where the *status quo* involves the absence of remedies, since the initial application of remedy continues to act, some physicians prefer to supply placebo (pilules of saccharum lactis = lactose = sac. lac. = S.L.). This is because it is believed that the patient will have difficulty in understanding that the original remedy is still working in his favour. This, however, in modern times is fairly inexcusable in most cases, unless the patient is fairly neurotic. Most patients are quite capable of understanding the matter of delayed effect, and to give them placebos is a breach of faith. In other instances, where there is a reasonable degree of organic change, a pathological remedy may be introduced, rather than give nothing at all. This method is often highly complementary to the action of the originally applied constitutional remedy, and accelerates the curative process.

Where, at the end of the first month, the patient is still in a phase of crisis, and this seems to have been going on for several weeks, it is best to discontinue the remedy, and wait for the improvement (healing) phase to commence. The patient will be the type who wishes to get better quickly, and he has 'grinned and born' the crisis, and continued the remedy without contacting you.

In rare instances, the healing crisis of the first month is not followed by an improvement phase, and the patient goes into an accelerated decline, even if the remedy has been discontinued. Sometimes, this accelerated decline occurs without any frank crisis, and the patient remains doggedly on the remedy, which must be stopped as soon as possible. This unfortunate situation occurs when we have failed to appreciate that the endocrine system of the patient is in a poor state, and we have caused it to overload, so to speak, by applying a deep-acting remedy.

This, obviously, should not happen if we appreciate the rules given previously with regard to where we should and should not apply such constitutional remedies. However, we must know what to do about this problem, should it arise. Fortunately, the 12c repetition method is not particularly aggressive, and, after stopping the remedy, the patient picks up in a few weeks. However, and this is most unusual with the use of lower potencies, it may be necessary to *antidote* the remedy.

The simplest manner in which this can be achieved is to insist that the patient drinks large amounts of coffee for several days, for coffee is the great antidote to many remedies. Alternatively, a specific antidote must be applied. Dr Gibson Miller's *Relationship of Remedies* will provide you with a list of suggested antidotes to the particular remedy that has caused problems.

You are required, however, to select the one most appropriate to the case at hand, and this must be determined by the symptomatology of the accelerated deterioration. The antidote might be given in a 12c, twice daily, until the patient improves, in which case it is stopped. Obviously, the best thing is to be careful in your application of remedies, and not to allow this sort of thing to happen!

Let us depart from these gloomy aspects of homoeopathy, especially since they are avoidable. Let us now consider how we might assess that a patient is being set on the curative path by our methods. In the first instance, he will tell you so. Whilst obvious, it is amazing how many physicians rely on special tests alone, which, after all, only give us a few dots in the clinical picture, in order to determine the state of the patient. The patient is a better judge in most cases. There should be both improvement in the presenting complaint, and an increase in general energy level. Often an improvement in general energy alone heralds improvement of the presenting complaint. The patient might say, 'Even though my joints still hurt, I feel a lot better in myself.' This is a good prognosticative sign, and indicates that our treatment is having a beneficial effect.

Apart from improvement of general energy and presenting complaint, we have other ways of telling that treatment is progressing satisfactorily. Whilst it is ridiculous to use special tests alone to assess the patient, their use is to be encouraged as supportive evidence. Additionally, we may utilize *Hering's Law* (Dr Hering was a famous pupil of Hahnemann's). This states:

'Cure occurs:

(a) From above downwards.

(b) From within outwards.

(c) In reverse chronological order.'

This means:

(a) 'From above downwards'. Cure progresses from the head towards the lower trunk; that is to say, head symptoms clear first. With regard to the extremities, cure spreads from shoulder to fingers, or hip to toes.

(b) 'From within outwards'. Cure progresses from more important organs (e.g. liver, endocrines) to less important organs (e.g. joints). That is to say, the function of vital organs is restored before those less important to life. The end result of this *'externalization'* of disease is often the production of a transient cutaneous rash; this fact having been mentioned previously with regard to the theory of Psora (psoric miasm).

(c) 'In reverse chronological order'. More recent symptoms and pathology will clear before old symptoms and pathology. The disease 'back-tracks', so to speak. After the more recent problems have been cleared, it is not at all uncommon for the patient to experience the transient recrudescence of old symptoms and pathology, which then disappear within a few weeks.

Hering's Law, which is also termed the *Law of Cure,* is the logical inverse of the way in which chronic disease progresses, both with regard to the patient himself and the ancestral history of disease. The *Law of Disease* might state:

'Disease progresses:

(a) From below upwards (hence, the progression of rheumatoid arthritis from small joints to large).

(b) From without inwards (hence, the suppression of skin disease may lead to asthma).

(c) In chronological order (which is obvious).'

Where the patient is being healed in accordance with the directives of Hering's Law we can assume that all is going well. The most important aspects of Hering's Law are 'from within outwards' and 'in reverse chronological order'. 'From above downwards' is the least important aspect, since whilst true of many cases, there are noteable exceptions. Where a skin disease has started on the head and progressed to the trunk, it is more likely to clear in reverse chronological order, viz. from below upwards. Nevertheless, exceptions are rare, and the newcomer may regard the Law to be generally applicable.

Generally speaking, increase in energy level and improvement in accordance with Hering's Law go hand in hand. Where the therapy is not producing changes in accord with the Law, there is also a failure to improve the level of general energy. Obviously, we must reconsider our therapeutic attack. In some cases, however, as with terminal cancer with gross auto-intoxication, the patient may be simply *incurable*. Whilst we must never declare any patient to be so without first making all possible attempts to heal, there comes a stage in these cases when we must content ourselves with making the residual lot of the patient more comfortable, and cast all healing attempts to the wind. These *incurable* cases are also the very cases which are sent on an accelerated downward path by the application of deep-acting remedies; a matter which has been discussed at some length.

The curative changes discussed with regard to Hering's Law

do not occur in the space of a few weeks. They occur in a period which ranges from several months to several years. Whilst we may have effectively reprogrammed the body with our therapy, the body still takes time to heal. There is a limit to the degree of acceleration of the healing process that we can expect. In this respect, both the homoeopathist and his patient must learn some patience. When all is going well, rest on your laurels, cautiously, of course, and preserve the *status quo*. Do not interfere and meddle with a successful therapeutic regime, by throwing in lots of extra remedies in the vain hope of curing the patient in a short time.

This is quite a different matter from the judicious modification of the therapeutic programme for good reason. Let us examine some of the reasons for modification of remedial therapy, and how we should act accordingly:

1. In some cases, especially those of children, the initially applied remedy is all that is needed to secure an effective cure. The remedy may have been withdrawn upon the occurrence of a healing crisis, or because the patient was rendered perfectly well, and deemed not to require further dosage. However, the occurrence of spontaneous acute disease requires the administration of pathological remedies in many instances. Should this occur whilst the patient is still taking the constitutional remedy, it is best to discontinue this remedy temporarily whilst we prescribe for the immediate acute illness. Generally, once the acute illness has passed, we may return to our previous constitutional remedy. Occasionally, the acute illness (e.g. measles) leaves the patient with a miasmic aftermath, which should be treated with an antimiasmatic remedy, before returning to constitutional therapy.

2. In many cases, after a few months, it becomes apparent that our constitutional remedy has achieved only a partial effect on the case. There are various distinctive varieties of this phenomenon, and it behoves us to describe both these and our appropriate actions:

(a) Having discontinued our remedy, with the patient rendered apparently 'cured', the case relapses. There is a remanifestation of the same disease complex. This may occur within a few weeks or several months of the discontinuation of the remedy. The same phenomenon of relapse also may occur where the patient has been maintained on the remedy because of progressive improvement. This may be due to:

(i) Failure to identify nutritional, and environmental modifying factors, and to eliminate them. An attempt must be made to identify these, and remove them where possible, after which the initial remedy may be reapplied as previously. However, where the environmental factors are strong and irremovable (e.g. work stress), it may be necessary to administer the same remedy in higher potency (see 2(a)(iii)). In many cases of hostile environment, the patient is obliged to continue taking constitutional remedies (usually intermittently), until such time as his circumstances change.

(ii) The remedy was acting in a pathological (peripheral) sense, rather than a constitutional. Cases that have a simple pathological expression (e.g. inflammatory mono-arthritis) often appear to clear up with a single pathological remedy, but, since the fundamental disease is still relatively unchallenged, they have a tendency to relapse. Upon careful review of the case, it will often be found that too much emphasis has been placed upon relatively recent aspects of mental and physical status. Our best action is to prescribe a new remedy based more firmly on the generals rather than these particulars. Alternatively, where this is problematical, due to a lack of well-defined generals, we might consider re-applying the same remedy in higher potency, e.g. 30c bd.

(iii) The selected potency has been too low to completely subdue the fundamental disease. Right remedy, wrong potency. This diagnosis is only valid if we are satisfied that the remedy is well-matched to the generals of the case, and that environmental and nutritional factors have not interfered. Our obligation is to re-apply the same remedy in higher potency. For this purpose, it is generally wise to proceed to a potency of 200c. There are various ways in which this may be given, but the safest way for the initiate is to give it as a *single dose* and await the results. The patient should be assessed after one month. Should this be fruitful, nothing else need be done, except to review the patient periodically. If relapse occurs again, then we must proceed to administer a single dose of 10M, and await the results. Similarly, we may be obliged to subsequently administer single doses of 50M or CM. Remember that, following the healing crisis, the progressive improvement of the patient obviates the need to prescribe a higher potency. Do not intervene if all is going well. If even a CM does not stabilize the case, it must be assumed that either a miasmatic factor is present, in which case an antimiasmatic remedy is needed, or that we have missed some nutritional or environmental factor of relevance. Where all attempts to stabilize the case result in failure, we may be committed to achieve stabilization by the intermittent use of these high potencies.

(b) Whilst the initially applied constitutional remedy is reasonably successful in clearing up various aspects of the case, it is not totally successful, and some problems remain:

(i) In the case of the patient with long-standing organic disease, you should suspect that a pathological prescription might be required. Whilst the constitutional remedy may have rendered the fundamental disease 'burnt out', it may not have the therapeutic range to cope with all peripheral changes. Therefore, a new prescription based on the particulars of the residual problems should be issued. In some instances, provided the remedies are compatible, it is possible to continue the basic constitutional remedy alongside the pathological remedy.

(ii) The selected constitutional remedy may be only attacking part of the fundamental disease complex. It is a *partial match*. It is better to reconsider the original generals of the case and attempt to find a better *similimum*. However, if this cannot be achieved, the case is best treated with the original remedy, plus various pathological remedies. Alternatively, a miasmic factor may be present for which an antimiasmatic remedy is required. The identification of miasmatic factors is discussed later, and the way in which we attack them. It is not always feasible to find a general constitutional remedy that will simultaneously remove miasms. However, once the miasmic factor has been subdued by the appropriate antimiasmatic remedy, the original remedy may be re-used with greater efficacy.

(iii) Lack of patience on the part of the practitioner, often provoked by a patient determined to get well fast. Often the remedy is working perfectly well, but improvement is slow. Both practitioner and patient must await the outcome, even if this means observing the patient over many months.

(c) Whilst the initially applied constitutional remedy is reasonably successful in clearing up the majority of the original aspects of the case, *new* symptoms arise:

(i) Many instances of the appearance of 'new' symptoms are, in actuality, in accordance with the third part of Hering's Law. They are the re-occurrence of *old* symptoms in reverse chronological order. Careful interrogation of the patient with regard to his past history often confirms this idea. The remedy, therefore, will be judged as appropriate to the case, and the *status quo* maintained. In many cases, these old symptoms spontaneously disappear, their occurrence being only 'symbolic'. In some, however, the case appears to get stuck. Whilst generally improved, the patient is unable to rid himself of this new occurrence of old symptomatology. In this instance, the prescription of a pathological remedy based upon the particulars of the new symptomatology will unstick the case. Where particularly obstinate, the presence of a miasm may be suspected, and an antimiasmatic remedy must be administered. Alternatively, a new constitutional remedy, based upon the generals of the case plus the new particulars, must be sought.

(ii) The constitutional remedy is proving itself. The patient, being particularly sensitive to the action of the remedy, generates new symptoms in accordance with those to be found in the *materia medica* with regard to the results of original provings of the remedy on healthy human volunteers. In this instance, there is to be found no evidence of the symptom in the past history of the patient. Consultation of *materia medica* will usually establish that the symptom has been experienced in the past during experimental proving. These proving symptoms are generally of little consequence, and rapidly disappear when the remedy is discontinued. Sometimes, with subsequent re-application of the same remedy, they do not become remanifest. Proving symptoms may occur with any remedy, irrespective of its depth of action, provided the patient is sensitive to it.

(iii) In some instances, new symptoms arise that cannot be classified as either 'old symptoms' or proving symptoms. These arise in accordance with the second part of Hering's Law: 'Cure occurs from within outwards'. They also may be regarded as detoxification symptoms in some cases. They may take the form of nasal catarrh, diarrhoea, or cutaneous rash. They indicate that the remedy is working correctly. Handling of the case proceeds along the lines described under 2(c)(i) as for the re-occurrence of old symptoms.

42.

Are Drugs and Homoeopathic Remedies Compatible?

The question is often raised as to whether allopathic drugs and homoeopathic remedies are compatible, or not? It has already been stated that drugs are suppressive in that they not only affect the destructive components of pathology, but they also affect the healing process itself. By contrast, homoeopathic remedies act by encouraging the latter.

On the face of it, they would seem to be totally incompatible, since they work in opposite directions on the healing process. Whilst it would be pleasant for all our patients to arrive for homoeopathic consultation without taking drugs, this, however, is often not the case. Should we immediately throw away the asthmatic's inhaler, which has been his lifeline for several years? Should we immediately deprive the grossly hypertensive patient of his antihypertensives, given to him after a stroke? Of course not! This would be foolish, irresponsible, and dangerous! Whereas, in the case of mild chronic disease, the abandonment of drug therapy can be instituted almost immediately, in the more serious cases it is not feasible.

Are we, therefore, as homoeopathists unable to consider treating these major cases? It would be a poor subject of ours if we were to accept such a defeatist attitude. In the first place, the institution of sound nutritional (and environmental) measures will often be of such assistance that the patient may reduce the level of drug therapy. Thus, the asthmatic with food allergy may benefit from the exclusion of the offending foods from the diet, the rheumatoid arthritic may benefit by the reduction of meat intake, and so on. Secondly, the power of remedies is such that they are frequently capable of over-riding the suppression of healing caused by drugs. Whilst the action of the remedy is somewhat inhibited by that of the drug, it is, nevertheless, not totally nullified. This, of course, depends to some degree on the nature of the drug in question. Steroids are particularly suppressive of healing, as all physicians realize. However, it is my personal experience that remedies may act beneficially, to some degree, even in the face of steroids. As the patient improves under our nutritional and medicinal therapy, so we may gradually withdraw the patient from conventional drugs. Whilst patients undergoing conventional drug therapy are slower to improve, improve they can!

43.

Antimiasmatic Remedies

A *miasm* may be defined as the persistent pathological after-math of infectious disease. A miasm may be either inherited or acquired. More than one miasm may be active in the same individual. Remedies that act against fundamental miasmatic disease are termed *antimiasmatic remedies*.

Whilst the infective origin of *inherited* miasms has been disputed by some authorities, the existence of miasms in general as *clinical syndromes* has not. That is to say, they represent clinically defineable physiological abnormalities, or particular types of constitutional trait.

It is often possible to infer the presence of one or more miasms from the details of the initial case history. In other instances, the presence of a miasm is deduced by the type of symptomatology that develops after remedial treatment has progressed for some time. As cure occurs in reverse chronological order, the 'new' symptoms that evolve may exhibit a pattern consistent with a particular miasmatic syndrome. Alternatively, failure of the case to respond to well-selected constitutional remedies of a general type may imply the presence of a miasmatic syndrome, which we may have failed to recognize at the outset.

Since the action of an initially applied general constitutional remedy may be so broad as to cover miasmatic syndromes, the use of antimiasmatic remedies is relegated to a secondary position in most cases. That is to say, even if the miasmatic base is identifiable in the initial history, we usually await the therapeutic outcome of the general constitutional prescription, before considering the application of an antimiasmatic remedy, for the application of the latter may be unnecessary. This is the surest course for the beginner. However, as experience is gained, it will become readily apparent that in certain situations it is permissible to apply an antimiasmatic remedy at the outset of the case. These are cases in which a particular miasmatic syndrome forms a dominant and well-defined aspect of the case history (e.g. a past history of severe reaction to smallpox vaccination).

Alternatively, there are cases where the particular type of pathology manifest shows a regular, though not necessarily absolute, correspondence with a particular miasm (e.g. many cases of enlarged adenoids in children are associated with a tuberculous miasm).

The miasms to be discussed are:

1. Psora.
2. Syphilitic miasm.
3. Sycosis (which includes Vaccinosis).
4. Tuberculous miasm.
5. Miasms following acute infections.

Psora is the miasmatic syndrome that is believed to arise from the suppression of infective skin disease. Whilst generally seen in its inherited form, its acquired origin may be determinable in the history of the patient. There may, for example, be an apparently spontaneous disappearance of herpes genitalis, reappearing in later life in the guise of cancer of the cervix.

The relentless suppression of any skin disease, infective or otherwise, with potent topical agents may force the fundamental disease to seek inward expression, and thus produce, in an artificial manner, the syndrome of Psora. Thus, eczema, an inherited psoric disease in its own right, may be converted to asthma by the injudicious use of steroid creams. The inherited psora is compounded in its expression by the acquisition of an artificial psoric component.

As a clinical syndrome, Psora is recognizable by the following features:

(a) Tendency to cutaneous or mucosal lesions (rashes, and catarrh of any mucosa).

(b) Periodicity of manifestation of cutaneous, mucosal, or serous disease.

(c) Alternation of the above lesions between themselves, or between the above lesions and those of internal organs or the psyche.

(d) Great susceptibility to parasitic infestation, or fungal infection (e.g. intestinal worms, thrush).

(e) Delayed recovery after acute or acute-on-chronic disease.

(f) Failure to respond satisfactorily to apparently well-selected general constitutional or pathological remedies.

Certain remedies exhibit a therapeutic correspondence to the syndrome of Psora in a marked manner. These so-called *antipsoric remedies* include: *Arsenicum album, Calcarea carbonica, Lycopodium,* and *Sulphur*. There are many others. You will recall that the remedies mentioned were discussed in connection with general constitutional therapy. Indeed, in many cases, Psora is subdued by the action of the general constitutional remedy alone. In those cases, however, where the cure has become obstructed, and the psoric miasm is identifiable as a clinical syndrome, then an antipsoric remedy must be subsequently introduced to unblock the case. Since there are in fact many possible alternatives, this selection may be difficult for the inexperienced. The whole matter is simplified, however, if the remedy *Sulphur* is used *to clear* the case, for *Sulphur* is the greatest of the antipsorics, and will unlock many a difficult case.

Hence, *a single dose* of *Sulphur* 30 may be given as the only remedy in a particular month, in an attempt to clear the psoric component. This in itself may produce a secondary healing crisis, as indeed any antimiasmatic remedy can, and, particularly in the case of *Sulphur,* cutaneous eruption (e.g. boils, pimples) may occur transiently. Thereafter, it is often possible to successfully re-apply the originally useful remedies in a case, which then will act with renewed vigour. It is sometimes necessary to re-apply a single dose of *Sulphur* (in the potency range 6-200) at a later stage, if another obstruction to main-line treatment occurs. This may, in fact, be necessarily repeated several times.

Where eczema cases are concerned, it may be undesirable to induce a potent healing crisis, and the use of high potencies of *Sulphur* is to be discouraged. Here, a single dose of *Sulphur* 6x or 6c should be given as a trial of effect. Generally, any healing crisis that occurs is of a mild nature. Following the crisis phase, there will be an improvement phase, but, since the low potency is weak in effect when given as a single dose, the patient will then usually relapse. The time interval between the administration of the single dose and the onset of relapse (*not* the onset of crisis) should be carefully recorded by the patient. This will approximately indicate the time interval required for dose repetition of the potency of *Sulphur,* for such repetition is generally required to achieve maximal therapeutic effect. This time interval usually varies between three and ten days. The number of doses required also varies considerably from case to case, but six doses constitute a good average starting regime, remembering to warn the patient to discontinue the remedy if a potent crisis occurs.

Minor healing crises aside, the physician should continue the dose repetition as long as background improvement occurs with regard to the eczema, although it may be necessary to lengthen the interval between doses. This will be necessary if the healing crises increase in strength. In some cases, it may be necessary to continue the regime for several months. Once background improvement ceases, or the eczema is no longer apparent, the regime may be abandoned. However, in unstable cases, it may warrant repetition at a later date.

Whilst *Sulphur* is a general constitutional remedy in its own right with regard to some eczema cases, in many others it constitutes a principal antipsoric, and thus is often prescribed in eczema cases in general. However, it must be emphasized that *Sulphur* is not merely an eczema remedy, but a potent antipsoric with regard to most manifestations of Psora.

Whilst *Sulphur* is the principal antipsoric, its nosodal analogue *Psorinum* should not be forgotten. Where *Sulphur* has failed as an antipsoric, *Psorinum* (prepared from a vesicle of scabies) may be considered as an alternative. *Psorinum* tends to be active in chilly individuals, whereas *Sulphur* acts better on hot individuals. A single dose of *Psorinum* 200 may be given, and the results awaited over a month. *Psorinum* is weaker in action than *Sulphur,* and generally is not so predisposed to the generation of potent healing crisis. It is of particular service in unblocking obstinate cases of psoriasis. Both *Sulphur* and *Psorinum* are key remedies in the constitutional desensitization to allergens.

The *syphilitic miasm* is believed to be due to ancestral syphilis, being generally of the inherited type. As a clinical syndrome it is characterized by:

(a) Lax ligaments, with a tendency to recurrent sprains, dislocations, and prolapse of internal organs.

(b) Grossly asymmetrical development of bones, leading to scoliosis.

(c) Tendency to form exostoses.

(d) Thickening of skin and mucous membranes (e.g. ichthyosis, leucoplakia).

(e) Stony hard lymphatic and glandular lesions.

(f) Tendency to ulceration.

(g) Mental retardation, or perversion of the intelligence.

(h) Aggravation of symptoms between dusk and dawn.

(i) Amelioration by mountain air.

As with all homoeopathic syndromes, you will be unlikely to meet a case that corresponds exactly to all these features. However, you will encounter many cases that correspond in part, and lead you to suspect that the use of an antisyphilitic is required. From the newcomers point of view, the two most important remedies in this connection are the syphilitic nosode *Lueticum (Syphilinum),* and *Calcarea fluorica. Lueticum,* administered in a 30 potency once weekly, is of service in the treatment of bone pains, especially if worse in the dark hours. *Calcarea fluorica* 30, twice weekly, is often of service in the treatment of those individuals who suffer from scoliosis, recurrent sprains and dislocations, or fibrotic conditions, such as Dupuytren's contracture. It is also of use in the treatment of severe nodular mastitis. As with all deep-acting remedies, dosage should be discontinued if the patient begins to feel unwell on the therapy.

Sycosis is the miasm that is believed to follow gonorrhoea, and may be inherited or acquired. In its acquired form, it may also arise from vaccination (vaccinosis) or immunization, allergic reactions to drugs or insect bites, and chronic infective states.

The clinical syndrome of sycosis is characterized by:

(a) Generalized fluid retention.

(b) Chronic catarrh of the mucous membranes.

(c) Papillomatous cutaneous lesions.

(d) Slow and progressive development with lack of periodicity.

(e) Sensitivity to cold and damp conditions.

(f) Tendency to depression.

(g) Polyp formation.

In this connection, we shall mention three major remedies: *Thuja, Natrum sulph.,* and *Medorrhinum* (nosode of gonorrhoea). *Thuja* is a most potent remedy, and whilst often quoted as a major wart remedy, is more specifically of service in the treatment of the ill-effects of vaccination. Any patient who has received vaccination or immunization, and reacted to it badly, should receive a single dose of *Thuja* 30, in order to prevent the development of an acquired sycosis. This, as has been stated, is an insidious illness, and may not become readily apparent in gross pathological terms until many years after the causative event. When well-ensconced, *Thuja* 30 should be given in infrequent doses, usually no more than once monthly.

Vaccinosis has been implicated in the development of malignancy. *Natrum sulph.* 30, given in intermittent dosage (e.g. twice weekly) is often useful in preventing the ill-effects of cold and damp, as in many cases of arthritis. *Medorrhinum* 200, a few monthly doses, should be given, probably routinely, to all who have suffered from gonorrhoea in the past, in order to clear any residual sycotic miasm. The same remedy is of great service in the treatment of polyp cases. Here, the 200 may be given once every two weeks.

The *tuberculous miasm* may be inherited or acquired, and is believed to stem from tuberculous infection. As a clinical syndrome, it is characterized by:

(a) A strong familial history, or a personal history, of tuberculosis.

(b) Inability to gain weight, despite a reasonable appetite.

(c) Susceptibility to respiratory infections and asthma.

(d) Profuse sweating.

(e) Fatigue and pallor.

(f) Hypertrophy of tonsils, adenoids and cervical lymph nodes.

(g) Strong allergic tendency.

(h) Periodicity of symptoms (e.g. periodic headaches).

As in other miasmatic syndromes, general constitutional remedies, such as *Silicea* (which is also an antisycotic), and *Phosphorus,* can exhibit an antituberculous effect. Where, however, they have been incomplete in their coverage of the case, and the tuberculous miasm is suspected, it is useful to introduce a remedy of the *Tuberculinum* (tuberculous nosode) group. The principal members of this group are *Tuberculinum Koch,* and *Tuberculinum bovinum.*

The Koch variety is generally more useful, and, given in infrequent doses (no more than once monthly) of 200 potency, is often used in cases of infantile lymphoid hypertrophy, recurrent bronchitis and asthma. It is a potent remedy, and should not be repeated too often. The bovinum variety is better indicated when there is pronounced cervical lymphadenopathy. When treating asthmatic patients, great caution should be observed in the use of *any* tuberculous nosode, for there is always a risk of aggravating the respiratory condition. They should never, therefore, be used at the outset of treatment in the case of any severely incapacitated asthmatic patient.

Miasms following *acute infections* are probably more common than we may realize. The diagnosis is often clear-cut, in that we are often told that the patient 'has never been well since ... e.g. measles'. Our usual course of action is to give a few bi-weekly doses of the appropriate nosode, often in a potency of 30 or 200. Hence, the use of *Glandular fever nosode* for the aftermath of glandular fever, and *Morbillinum* for the aftermath of measles. Such an approach, however, sometimes fails. Should this happen, we are obliged to find the general constitutional remedy of the patient which matches the generals of the case *prior* to the onset of the acute illness. This is administered as for any other general constitutional remedy. By matching the remedy against the pre-acute constitution, we are, in effect, treating the susceptibility to miasmic development, rather than the outcome. We are treating more deeply than would be possible by taking the particulars of the acquired miasm into consideration, which essentially, would be a pathological prescription. Whilst it would be possible to treat the patient in this manner, the deeper approach is more swift.

44.

Pathological Remedies

Pathological remedies are those which act on the peripheral aspects of disease, rather than the fundamental. They are of service in the treatment of both acute and chronic illness. With regard to pathological remedies, we may talk in terms of three classes of action:

1. Pathotropism.
2. Organotropism.
3. Aetiotropism.

Pathotropism implies the affinity for particular types of pathological process. Hence, the use of the remedy *Ferrum phos.* in the early stages of acute inflammation throughout the body.

Organotropism implies the affinity for particular sites of disease, be they organs as such, or tissues. *Phosphorus,* for example, has an affinity for the lungs and the liver, covering a wide variety of pathologies, including bronchitis, pneumonia, viral hepatitis, and cirrhosis. With respect to joints, *Bryonia* is both organotropic, in that it has an affinity for these structures, and pathotropic, in that it corresponds to a particular type of inflammation within them.

Aetiotropism implies the affinity of remedies for illnesses brought on by particular events. These are those remedies prescribed on the basis of circumstantial *causation*. Hence, the use of *Aconite* in a variety of ailments brought on by sudden chilling, and the use of *Ignatia* in ailments brought on by loss of a loved one.

Pathological remedies by no means constitute a unique class of medicinal agents. Whereas some remedies, such as *Hecla lava* (lava from Mount Hecla), useful in the reduction of osteophytes, are restricted largely to the pathological sphere of action, others, such as *Phosphorus,* exhibit well-defined constitutional functions. Whilst *Phosphorus* is a constitutional remedy of great power in those cases where it matches the generals, it is a pathological remedy in those where it matches the particulars. Indeed, in those situations where the production of a potent healing crisis would be undesirable, and a potentially deep-acting remedy has been selected for its pathological correspondence, it is most important that the remedy does not match the generals to a significant degree. Certain instances of healing crisis ascribable to pathological prescription are probably due to the remedy having a correspondence in part to the constitution of the patient. This, however, occurs rarely.

It is not possible in an introductory work to list all the various possibilities with regard to pathological prescribing. The physician is referred to Clarke's *Prescriber,* and Boericke's *Materia Medica,* both rich sources of such information. However, I shall endeavour to give you some basic illustrations of pathological prescription in chronic disease.

In the treatment of *arthritis,* there are numerous pathological remedies, but three figure prominently: *Rhus tox., Bryonia* and *Perna can.* (Green-lipped New Zealand Mussel). Though all three are markedly organotropic to joints, prescription must be based on a careful analysis of the particulars, or failure will result. They are not to be prescribed 'willy nilly'. The specific indications are as follows:

(a) *Rhus tox.* Pains in joints worse on initial movement, and then improved by continued movement. A great remedy for 'stiffness', loosened by motion. Joints worse for damp, cold weather. Concomitant symptoms: great restlessness, especially at night.

(b) *Bryonia.* Hot, swollen joints, worse for *all* movement, and better for rest. Worse for hot weather. Concomitant symptoms: general fatigue, and general dryness of mucous membranes.

(c) *Perna can.* This is a relatively recent addition to the *materia medica,* whose properties are not so well-established as the more traditional remedies. Its principal indication, however, would seem to be degenerative arthritis of the first metatarso-phalangeal joint and hip, in the absence of any marked concomitant symptoms.

These points clearly indicate that the prescription of organotropic remedies is based upon more than this facility alone. The actual anatomical site of the disease, the nature of the pathological process, and the modalities may all be relevant to effective prescribing. Neither should concomitant symptoms be ignored in this respect, should they be present. At first sight, it might be thought that consideration of concomitants in pathological prescribing is to bring the generals of the case into the prescription, and thus indulge in constitutional therapy.

However, concomitant symptoms, mental or physical, are those which accompany the disorder, and were not present before its onset. They are, therefore, to be regarded as particulars of the case, rather than generals. That they fall outside the bounds of the conventional diagnostic category of the presenting complaint is utterly immaterial. They are true components of this disease. Hence, the physician must learn to ask more of his patient than those facts immediately related to his principal pathology, in order to establish a pathological prescription with efficacy.

In cases of chronic arthritis, both *Rhus tox.* and *Bryonia* are often prescribed in a 6 potency, bd. *Perna can.* is best prescribed in low potency, 3x or 6x, bd. *Rhus tox.* is also a potent eye remedy, and is of service in the treatment of Reiter's syndrome. In this connection, the 'bowel nosode' *Sycotic co.* should also be mentioned for its therapeutic value.

In eczema, we have *Graphites,* particularly suited to cases of weeping and cracking, and *Petroleum,* where the skin is worse in the winter months. In psoriasis, *Arsenicum album* and *Hydrocotyle asiatica* (Indian pennywort) figure prominently. In herpes genitalis, *Natrum mur., Sepia, Petroleum* and *Rhus venenata* (Poison-elder) are worthy of mention. All, of course, will have their own specific indications listed in the *materia medica.*

As a general rule, most pathological remedies are safely and effectively administered as a 6 potency, bd. Where 6 is unavailable, 12 or 30 potencies may be used in most instances. Certain pathological remedies, however, especially those prepared from endocrine products, are sufficiently potent to require repetition less frequently.

Thyroidinum 12 (prepared from the gland) given twice weekly, assists in the treatment of many hypertensive cases. *Nux vomica* 6, given bd, may be used in the treatment of intermittent arterial hypertension. *Crataegus* (Hawthorn berry), which is probably both a nutritional cardiac aid and a remedy in the usual homoeopathic sense, is given as Ø, 5 drops bd or tid in a little water. It is indicated in the damaged, failing, or irregular heart.

Sepia 6, bd, for a week or so prior to menstruation, alleviates many cases of premenstrual tension. *Magnesia phos.* is almost specific for menstrual colic, but may be required in a potency of 30-200 in order to produce great relief. Initially, it may be necessary to repeat it every $\frac{1}{2}$-1 hour. *Folliculinum* 12 (Oestrone), given as a single dose on the tenth day of each cycle, is used to treat a variety of menstrual and ovulatory problems.

An interesting group of remedies, commonly available from most pharmacies these days, are the so-called *tissue* salts of Dr Schussler. There are twelve in all:

Calc. fluor.	*Kali sulph.*
Calc. phos.	*Mag. phos.*
Calc. sulph.	*Nat. mur.*
Ferr. phos.	*Nat. phos.*
Kali mur.	*Nat sulph.*
Kali phos.	*Silicea.*

You will, I trust, recognise some of these remedies from our previous discussions. The term *tissue salts* stems from the unwarranted claim that they act as direct cell *nutrients,* when, in actuality, they are no more than homoeopathic remedies issued in low potency, generally 2x or 6x. At such low levels of potentization, they cannot, of course, have sufficient energy in most cases to act as constitutional remedies. This does happen occasionally, however, with the generation of a minor healing crisis. Essentially, they are selected as pathological remedies, and repeated as often as three times daily, or more frequently in the case of acute disease. Sometimes minor healing crisis will occur due to too frequent repetition for too great a period.

They are, however, very safe, and since many of your patients will have tried them for various complaints, often without knowledge of their homoeopathic origin, you should be familiar with them. You may even wish to experiment with them personally. Moreover, they are often put out as mixtures of several 'tissue salts', in order to simplify prescribing. One word of warning should be issued, however, with regard to dosage. Whilst the general rule for prescribing is that one tablet equals one dose, this may not be so in the case of some of the cheaper commercial preparations. Due to insufficient compression of the triturated material, up to four pills may be required to constitute a dose. For practical details of prescribing these low potency remedies, you are referred to *The Biochemic Handbook,* published by Thorsons.

You are by now aware of the ability of homoeopathic remedies to exert an action simultaneously on both the mental and the physical sphere. However, you will frequently come across cases with a very dominant mental factor. In these cases, it is not uncommon for classical remedies, selected on the basis of both the physical and mental aspects, to fail. This may be so even if those remedies were apparently well-chosen, and active at the constitutional level. They may either fail outright, which is rare, or the case will relapse and relapse, until all remedial applications would seem a hopeless waste of time, both to patient and physician.

The destructive effect of the psyche is so great as to prevent or undo any good work, or so it would seem. Hence, the case of eczema in an adult, where the disease represents an externalization of some deep emotional problem, and the subconscious will not relieve the body of its outlet. The psyche continually induces the recrudescence of fundamental disease, and its superficial manifestations.

Neither is psychotherapy necessarily the answer, although it is capable of inducing great improvement in many cases, for the patient may have neither the time nor the wish for it. Should we ourselves despair? Perhaps not, for there are further remedial measures available in such cases.

Considering the mind as an organ in its own right, we must apply psycho-organotropic remedies. Whilst classical psychotropic remedies, such as *Ignatia* and *Pulsatilla* (usually in 12 potency, bd) may be tried, they themselves may fail. A more fruitful approach is to use an important group of therapeutic agents, known as the *Bach flower remedies*. The flower remedies and their principal indications are as follows:

1. AGRIMONY. Mental torture behind a brave face.
2. ASPEN. Fears of unknown origin.
3. BEECH. Intolerant and precise.
4. CENTAURY. Timid and weak-willed.
5. CERATO. Doubt of own ability, and seeks advice from all and sundry.
6. CHERRY PLUM. Fear of losing control and reason.
7. CHESTNUT BUD. Failure to learn from past errors.
8. CHICORY. Selfish and possessive.
9. CLEMATIS. Vacant and indifferent.
10. CRAB APPLE. Self-dislike and feels unclean.
11. ELM. Sense of inadequacy in the face of responsibilities.
12. GENTIAN. Easily discouraged.
13. GORSE. Utter despair.
14. HEATHER. Totally self-interested.
15. HOLLY. Envious or jealous.
16. HONEYSUCKLE. Dwells on the past.
17. HORNBEAM. Mental and physical fatigue.
18. IMPATIENS. Impatient and nervous.

19. LARCH. Lack of self-confidence.
20. MIMULUS. Fears of known things.
21. MUSTARD. 'Endogenous' depression.
22. OAK. Overworks, but struggles on.
23. OLIVE. Total exhaustion.
24. PINE. Guilt 'complex'.
25. RED CHESTNUT. Over-concern for others.
26. ROCK ROSE. Terror or panic (useful after nightmare).
27. ROCK WATER. Rigidity of outlook and self-denial.
28. SCLERANTHUS. Indecisive.
29. STAR OF BETHLEHEM. Shock.
30. SWEET CHESTNUT. Great anguish.
31. VERVAIN. Perfectionistic and over-anxious.
32. VINE. Ruthlessness.
33. WALNUT. Over-sensitive to outside influences.
34. WATER VIOLET. Aloof.
35. WHITE CHESTNUT. Persistent, unwanted thoughts.
36. WILD OAT. Indecision about future plans.
37. WILD ROSE. Apathetic resignation.
38. WILLOW. Resentment.
39. RESCUE REMEDY. Discussed in acute disease section.

The flower remedies are generally supplied in liquid form, and do not carry a potency symbol. The dose is usually three drops tid, except in acute situations, where the remedy may be repeated very frequently.

The flower remedies have not only the virtue of minimal toxicity, but also the ability to match many common psychological problems. They are readily applied to the general practice situation. Whilst it is the fashion with some practitioners to issue mixtures of up to six remedies, in order to cover the case, this is not to be encouraged, for there is a risk of one remedy antidoting another. This risk is totally eliminated by taking your time over the case, and selecting a single remedy that best matches the mental status. At any rate, never mix more than two remedies in one prescription.

In selecting Bach flower remedies, the physical components of the disease are ignored in favour of a detailed analysis of the psyche. It must be admitted that this in itself has some psychotherapeutic effect. Where the physical problems stem from disorder of the psyche, they too will clear up with an appropriate psychotropic remedy. For further details, the physician is referred to *Handbook of the Bach Flower Remedies* by P. M. Chancellor (C. W. Daniel).

Another interesting group of modern pathological remedies are those prepared from allergens. Hence, the use of *House-dust mite,* 30, *Mixed pollens* 30, and *Lac vaccinum* 30 (cow's milk) in the treatment of specific allergic states. They may be used to prevent reaction, and, in some instances, may effectively cure the particular sensitivity. They do not, however, in general have any significant effect on fundamental disease, which may become remanifest as the acquisition of a new allergy.

45.

Final Summary

You are now coming to the end of your initial journey into a revolutionary new field of medicine. Do not be put off by its apparent complexity, for, rather like a game of chess, it is founded on very simple and logical principles. The principles are straightforward, the ramifications complex.

Let us quickly review the methods by which we treat cases of chronic disease:

1. Nutritional modification.
2. Environmental modification (where possible).
3. General constitutional prescription.
4. Antimiasmatic prescription.
5. Pathological prescription (utilizing the organotropic, pathotropic, and aetiotropic affinities of remedies).

It would be surprising if this did not seem a trifle overwhelming to the initiate. Indeed, it might appear to be totally unmanageable in the average practice situation. This, however, is far from the truth. After all, you are neither required, nor is it appropriate, to apply all these measures simultaneously on any particular case.

The time is June, and a young man enters your surgery with severe hay-fever. Your responsibility is to alleviate his suffering primarily, not to cure him of his disease. You must give him a pathological prescription, which may be *Sabadilla* (Cevadilla seed), *Euphrasia offic.*, *Allium cepa* (Onion), *Arsenicum album,* and so on, according to the correspondence of his particulars with the contents of the *materia medica,* or *therapeutic index.* You may even consider giving him potentized *Mixed pollens* or *Mixed grasses;* orally, of course. If your initial prescription fails, this is not to be regarded as a failure of homoeopathy, but a failure on your part to determine the appropriate remedial action. Do not give up, but represcribe. Also consider giving the patient Vitamin C daily, to assist in detoxification, and thus render your remedy more therapeutically active. Manage the case in this manner until the end of the season, at which time you should take the case in some detail.

Now you may indulge in your more curative work, to subdue the fundamental disease of origin. There is often little point in commencing the use of deep-acting remedies in the hay-fever season, for the toxicity of the patient will tend to negate their action. Moreover, as I have said, the patient merely seeks relief at that time, without side-effects, of course. Over many months, you will apply general constitutional therapy, and antimiasmatic therapy. How will you know, however, that your remedies are having some effect before the onset of the next hay-fever season? Because well-chosen, deep-acting remedies tend to produce constitutional disturbance, or healing crisis. If your remedy has zero effect on the patient, you may assume that the remedy is probably ill-chosen.

The next hay-fever season comes. The patient reappears. Your face drops, for he still has hay-fever. You glance through your records. His general constitutional remedy was *Phosphorus,* which gave him transient headaches and a mild epistaxis. His antiasmatic remedies were *Sulphur,* which gave him some transient pimples on his face, and *Tuberculinum Koch,* which produced a bout of hay-fever like symptoms out of season. 'But my symptoms are a lot less than they were before,' he says, 'and the pollen count is very high!'

So, back to Vitamin C and *Sabadilla,* or whatever, for the rest of the season. At the end of the season, repeat the constitutional therapy. Always repeat those remedies that gave healing crisis previously. Only use new constitutional remedies if the originals fail to induce constitutional reaction on their second application.

Next season, he reappears. No hay-fever, just a carbuncle on his neck, which you proceed to treat with *Tarentula cubensis.*

It is sometimes remarked that homoeopathy is slow. This is true with regard to some chronic diseases, especially if there has been marked organic change. But this is much better than no cure at all, which is usually the case with many allopathic treatments. In general, patients should expect to undergo therapy for a period of 6-24 months, before they are stabilized, after which time they can often discontinue all medicinal therapy, whilst maintaining any nutritional therapy deemed necessary. With regard to acute disease, homoeopathy is amazingly swift and effective. In an infective illness, the remedy often works faster than the antibiotic. Neither is it deterred by a viral presence.

One of the greatest problems for the newcomer to homoeopathy is the great variety of ways in which it is possible to view any particular case. Indeed, two experienced practitioners may disagree on the identity of the initial remedy. This in itself should not cause discouragement, for rather like chess, there are many possible moves, and many different ways of winning the game. If anything, it is a tribute to the great flexibility of the subject with regard to the curative process. There are many paths that lead to our goal.

A final tip. When you are unable to decide with which remedy to follow on, refer to Dr Gibson Miller's *Relationship of Remedies*. Look up the last remedy that had some clinical effect (always ignore a remedy that has had no effect whatsoever). Examine the sections marked 'Complements', and 'Remedies That Follow Well'. Commit yourself to using one of these, choosing that remedy best matched to the case at hand. When using this book, it must be said that the section marked 'Duration', which refers to the duration of action of remedies, can be largely ignored, for this matter depends on the individuality of the patient, and the potency of the selected remedy.

46.

Test Paper

A final set of questions. There may be several correct answers to each question:

1. Which of the following statements is true with regard to exclusion diets in cases of suspected food allergy?

(a) They should be abandoned if the patient does not improve within two weeks of commencement.

(b) They should be abandoned if the patient's condition worsens within two weeks of commencement.

(c) They are pointless if the results of skin testing are negative.

(d) They should be continued for at least one month.

2. A patient presents with chronic constipation, despite a satisfactory intake of dietary fibre, generalized mild fluid retention, and muscular cramps. Which of the following diagnoses should be considered?

(a) Aluminium sensitivity.

(b) Zinc deficiency.

(c) Cow's milk allergy.

(d) Vitamin B^6 (pyridoxine) deficiency.

3. Multiple white spots on the nails may be due to:

(a) Calcium deficiency.

(b) Zinc deficiency.

(c) Silicea constitution.

(d) Intermittent fasting.

4. A lady of 65 wishes you to prescribe homoeopathic treatment for her generalized osteoarthritis. Whilst she takes no medication for her arthritis, you discover that she has severe congestive heart failure, for which she is taking digoxin and a diuretic. Her generals reveal that her general constitutional type corresponds to the remedy *Phosphorus*. What should you do?

(a) Take her off all her drugs.

(b) Assess her nutritional status.

(c) Prescribe *Phosphorus*.

(d) Prescribe a pathological remedy.

5. A timid young lady enters your surgery. She is tearful, and

her face is covered with urticaria, which she has experienced intermittently for some years, and for which no apparent cause has been found. She also complains of a persistent bland vaginal discharge, and greenish chronic nasal catarrh. What is her most likely general constitutional remedy?

    (a) *Pulsatilla.*
    (b) *Phosphorus.*
    (c) *Natrum mur.*
    (d) *Calcarea carb.*

6. Which of the following remedies is the principal opponent of the miasm of Vaccinosis?

    (a) *Tuberculinum Koch.*
    (b) *Silicea.*
    (c) *Thuja.*
    (d) *Sepia.*

7. Which of the following characterize the miasm of Psora?

    (a) Alternation.
    (b) Periodicity
    (c) Susceptibility to fungal infection.
    (d) Fluid retention.

8. Which of the following remedies may be considered as antipsoric?

    (a) *Hecla lava.*
    (b) *Sulphur.*
    (c) *Euphrasia.*
    (d) *Psorinum.*

9. Which of the following is useful in the pathological treatment of premenstrual syndome?

    (a) *Sepia.*
    (b) *Sabadilla.*
    (c) *Mag. phos.*
    (d) Vitamin B^6 (pyridoxine).

10. Which miasmatic syndrome is characterized by slow and progressive development, fluid retention, and the presence of multiple cutaneous papillomata?

    (a) Psora.
    (b) Sycosis.
    (c) Syphilitic miasm.
    (d) Tuberculous miasm.

11. Of which of the following is the sensation 'burning relieved by heat' a characteristic symptom?

    (a) *Sulphur.*
    (b) *Phosphorus.*

(c) *Arsenicum album.*

(d) *Natrum mur.*

12 Which of the following may be regarded as characteristic of the Phosphoric constitution?

(a) Headaches brought on by thundery weather.

(b) Clairvoyance.

(c) Bruising tendency.

(d) Tall, thin morphology.

13. Which of the following should you associate with the syndrome of scoliosis, multiple exostoses, and recurrent sprains?

(a) *Calcarea carb.*

(b) *Silicea.*

(c) *Lycopodium.*

(d) *Calcarea fluor.*

14. Which of the following is true with regard to the remedy *Tuberculinum Koch?*

(a) It is useful in many cases of adenoidal hypertrophy.

(b) It is generally repeated twice daily for several weeks.

(c) It is seldom valuable in potencies above 6c.

(d) It is useful in many cases of asthma.

ANSWERS:

1d, 2a, 3bcd, 4bd, 5a, 6c, 7abc, 8bd, 9ad, 10b, 11c, 12abcd, 13d, 14ad.

Useful Addresses

Homoeopathic pharmacies:
Ainsworth's Homoeopathic Pharmacy
38 New Cavendish Street
London W1M 7LH
Tel: 01-935 5330/01-486 0459.

Nelson's Homoeopathic Pharmacy
73 Duke Street
Grosvenor Square
London W1M 6BY
Tel: 01-629 3118/9.

Boericke and Tafel Inc.,
1011 Arch Street
Philadelphia
PA 19107
USA

Homoeopathic organizations:
British Homoeopathic Association
27A Devonish Street
London W1N 1RJ
Tel: 01-935 2163.

Faculty of Homoeopathy
The Royal London Homoeopathic Hospital
Great Ormond Street
London WC1N 3HR
Tel: 01-837 3091 Extn: 72

Index

ABC, 29, 30, 35, 37, 40, 57
abscess, breast, 22
    dental, 48
absorption, inadequate intestinal, 69, 70
Acidum nitricum, 39
Acidum phosphoricum, 38
acne vulgaris, 23, 77
Aconite (Aconitum napellus), 27, 29, 35, 37, 38, 40, 49, 145
addiction, 84
adults, chronic disease in, 75, 76
aetiotropism, 145
aggravation, chemical, 126
    homoeopathic, see *healing crisis.*
alcohol, excesses of, 78
alcohol-water, 11
alcoholism, 84
alfalfa, 81, 101
allergy, 101
    desensitization in, 141
    food, 61, 70, 71, 92-8
    role of tuberculous miasm in, 66
Allium cepa, 152
allopathy, 10, 102
Alumina, 90
aluminium sensitivity, 70, 90, 91
anaesthetic, general, somnolence after, 52
angina pectoris, 47
Anthracinum, 48
antibiotics, ill-effects of, 39
antidote, necessity to, 129, 130
Antimonium crudum, 48
Antimonium tartaricum, 31, 38, 40
antipsoric, 66, 139-141
Apis mellifica, 31, 48, 53
Argentum nitricum, 43
Arnica montana, 18, 19, 49, 52, 125
Arsenicum album, 26, 31, 50, 110, 112, 113, 116, 117, 124, 139, 147, 152
arthritis, 146
    damp induced, 73
    diet in, 83
    inflammatory, 93
asthma, 31, 93, 103, 143
    role of tuberculous miasm in, 66
aversions, 112

Bach flower remedies, 31, 149, 150
Baptisia, 37, 40
barbecues, 79
barley, 101

Belladonna, 22, 29, 30, 31, 40, 48
benoxaprofen, 114
Biochemic Handbook. The, 148
blebs, 53
boils, 31, 48, 140
    recurrent, 48
bones, contused, 49
    nocturnal pain in, 142
Borax, 39
bowel, obstructed, 50
bran, 77, 78
breasts, engorgement of, 52
bronchitis, acute, 31, 37, 38
Bryonia, 22, 38, 145-147
burns, 16, 18, 31, 100

cabbage, 81
Cactus grandiflorous, 47
Calcarea carbonica, 35, 111-113, 117, 139
Calcarea fluorica, 74, 142, 148
Calcarea phosphorica, 118, 148
Calendula, 16, 18, 31, 51, 52
camphor, 17
cancer, 88, 101, 142
    cervical, 139
Cantharis, 50, 53
Carbo vegetabilis, 47
carbohydrates, refined, 70, 77
carbuncle, 48
cardamom, 81
case, 'burnt out', 106, 107, 127, 128
    clearing of, 140
catarrh, 61, 93
Caulophyllum, 52
causation, 26, 27, 145
cellulitis, 48
Chamomilla, 30, 101
chicken-pox, 40, 42
children, chronic disease in, 75, 76
    hyperactive, 70, 93
chilling, sudden, 27
China (Cinchona officinalis), 10, 47, 50
Cocculus indicus, 43
coffee, 16, 19, 129
cold, common, 37, 42
colic, 50
    menstrual, 50, 147
colitis, 93
collapse, sudden, 47
Collinsonia canadensis, 51
Colocynthis, 50
compatibility of drugs and remedies, 136, 137
Concise Repertory of Homoeopathic Medicines, A, 55

conjunctivitis, 16, 19
constipation, 80
    of pregnancy, 51
constitution, alterable aspects of, 112
    change of, 111, 112
    fixed aspects of, 112
    relevance in acute prescribing of, 23
contraceptives, oral, 100
contracture, Dupuytren's, 74, 142
'corpse reviver, homoeopathic', 47
corroboration, clinical, 54
Crataegus, 16, 147
Crohn's disease, 93
croup, infantile, 38
Cuprum metallicum, 90
cure, 61, 72-4
cure, the grape, 87
cyst, calcified, 74
cystitis, acute, 50

dampness, ill-effects of, 73
dandelion, 101
desiccation, 13, 17
desires, 112
detoxification, 87, 104, 107, 125, 135, 152
diarrhoea, chronic, 93
diet, exclusion, 94-8
    high-fibre, 78
    low-fibre, 78
    sensible basic, 77-9
dilution, scales of, 11-13
    serial, 11
disease, acute, reasons for treating, 21
    cardiovascular, 99, 100
    chronic, acute illness during treatment of, 132
    chronic, nature of, 61-3
    chronic, objectives of therapy in, 102
    fundamental, 61-7, 73, 74, 97, 102-104, 106
    incurable, 131
    infective, action of remedies in, 21
    psychosomatic, 150
    reversibility of, 68
    stereotyping of, 22
disorganization, anatomical, 74
dosage, 16
    repetition of, in acute disease, 34
drainage, 107
drainer, 125
Drosera, 40

drug rash, 39
drugs, allopathic, 102, 103
  side-effects of, 103
  withdrawal of, 87, 88
eczema, 16, 66, 77, 93, 140, 141,
  147, 149
  infected, 48
  use of steroids in, 103
eggs, 77
elbow, tennis, 49
endocrines, dysfunction of, 67
energy, general, 105, 106, 130,
  131
environment, 68,69
epidemics, 27
  preventative remedies in, 27
epistaxis, acute, 35
Eupatorium perfoliatum, 37
Euphrasia officinalis, 16, 18, 19,
  40, 152
eustachian catarrh, subacute, 36
examinations, fear of, 43
exercise, 84, 85
externalization, 130, 135
eye-strain, 49

factors, modifying, 63-71, 72, 73
faint, simple, 47
fat, 77
fear, states causing, 29
Ferrum phosphoricum, 35, 37,
  145, 148
fever, 29, 30, 35
fevers, specific infectious, 40, 41
fibrosis, 100
figs, syrup of, 81
flatulence, 81, 82
flour, 77
Folliculinum, 147
food, toxic contamination of, 70,
  77
fracture, non-union of, 49
fright, 27
fruit, 78
frying, 78, 79
furuncles, see boils

gall-bladder, disease of, 81
garlic, 35, 37, 39, 101
gastric irritation, 31, 50
gastroenteritis, acute, 31, 50
Gelsemium, 37, 38, 43, 118
genes, role of, in disease, 63-7
generals, 109-115, 128
genus epidemicus, 27
German measles, 40
gingivostomatitis, acute herpetic,
  41
glandular fever, 33, 40, 144
Glandular fever nosode, 33, 40,
  143
gluten sensitivity, 78, 96
gonorrhoea, 142, 143
gout, 104
granulocytosis, 33
Graphites, 16, 118, 147
grief, 27
Gunpowder, 31, 48

haemorrhoids, 16, 51, 80
Hahnemann, Dr C.F.S., 9
Hamamelis virginica, 16
Handbook of the Bach Flower
  Remedies, 150

hay-fever, 101, 152, 153
headaches, 93
healing crisis, 45, 51, 87, 96, 97,
  104-107, 125-129, 140, 141,
  146, 148, 153
heart, failing, 147
Hecla lava, 145
Hepar sulphuris, 22, 35, 38, 48
Hering's Law, see Law of Cure
herpes genitalis, 139, 147
  labialis, 48
  zoster, 48
home remedy kits, 28-32
homoeopathicity, 21
homoeopathy, etymology of, 10
homoeopathy, therapeutic speed
  of, 153
honey, 77
House-dust mite, 151
Hughes, Dr Richard, 10
Hydrocotyle asiatica, 147
Hypericum, 52
hypertension, 78, 100, 147
hypertrophy, chronic lymphoid,
  143
hypnosis, 98
hypoglycaemia, 84-6, 100

Ignatia, 27, 118, 145, 149
illness, mental, 31
immunization, homoeopathic, 42
  miasmata following, 66, 67
impetigo, 48
index, therapeutic, 53, 54
indigestion, 81, 82
infarction, myocardial, 47
infection, predisposition to
  recurrent, 30, 31
influenza, 37, 42
Influenzinum Co., 37, 42
inheritance, Lamarckian, 64
instructions to patients, 19
internalization, 64-6, 103
investigation, pathological, 33,
  130
Ipecacuanha, 27, 38, 40, 51

Jaborandi, 40
juice 'fast', 39

Kali. bichromicum, 38
Kali, carbonicum, 51
Kali, muriaticum, 36, 148
kelp, 51, 71, 100

labour, 52
Lac caninum, 52
Lac vaccinum, 151
Lachesis, 48, 118
lactation, 52, 71
lactose, 11, 15, 129
latency, 64, 73
Latrodectus mactans, 47
Law of Cure (Hering's Law),
  130-132, 134, 135
  Disease, 131
  Similars, 9, 65, 114
  Similars, corollary of The, 116
laxatives, 81
lecithin, 100
Lueticum (Syphilinum), 142
lumbago, 49
  of pregnancy, 51

Lycopodium, 13, 112, 113, 119,
  139

Magnesia phosphorica, 50, 147,
  148
Magnetis polus australis, 48
malaria, 10
mastitis, nodular, 142
materia medica, 53-6, 113, 114
measles, 23, 40, 42
Medorrhinum, 142
mentals, 110-112
Mercurius solubilis, 22, 30, 35,
  40, 41, 44, 45, 119, 120
message, pharmacological, 11, 13
miasm, 133-135, 138-144
  definition of, 65
  following acute infective
    illness, 143, 144
  prevention of, 65
  syphilitic, 141, 142
  tuberculous, 139, 143
migraine, 61, 84, 93, 94, 96
mind and body, integral nature
  of, 112
Mixed grasses, 152
Mixed pollens, 151, 152
modalities, 113, 114
  definition of, 26
  general, 112
Morbillinum, 40, 42, 65, 144
morphology, 113
multiple sclerosis, 93
mumps, 40, 42
muscles, fatigued, 49
  pulled, 49
Myristica, 48

Natrum muriaticum, 37, 48, 110,
  120, 142, 147, 148
Natrum sulphuricum, 73, 148
neuralgia, migrainous facial, 93
nipples, cracked, 52
nosode, bowel, 147
  definition of, 30
  preventative action of, 42
  use of, in miasmatic case, 65
nutrition, inadequate, 68-71
Nux vomica, 14, 31, 37, 50, 51,
  110, 111, 120

occupation, 110, 111
oil, cod-liver, 100
olive, 81
operation, fear of, 43
Opium, 52
organizations, homoeopathic,
  157
Organon, The, 9, 72
organotropism, 54, 145
orthopaedics, 49
Oscillococcinum, 30, 37, 40, 42
osteoarthritis, 70, 74, 99, 100
otitis media, acute, 35
  serous, 93

Parotidinum, 40,42
particulars, 109, 113, 114, 128
pathogenesis, 54
pathotropism, 145
peppermint, 101
Perna canalicula, 146, 147

Pertussin, 40, 42
Petroleum, 43, 147
pharmacies, homoeopathic, 158
Phosphorus, 34, 37, 38, 54, 110,
　113, 114, 120,143, 145, 153
Phytolacca, 22, 40
pica, 112
placebo, 129
Pocket Manual of Homoeopathic
　Materia Medica, 54, 55, 146
poisoning, 54, 126
poisons, preparation of, 13
polychrest, 76
　definition of, 34
polyp, 142, 143
polypharmacy, 29, 45, 148, 150
postinfluenzal states, 38
potency, 12
　destruction of, 17, 19, 20
　selection of, 124-126
potentization, 12
predisposition, pathological, 113
pregnancy, 51, 52, 71
　nutritional supplements in, 51
Prescriber, The, 23-25, 53, 54,
　146
prescribing, methods of, 44-6
proving, 54, 114, 135
Psora, 66, 130, 139-141
psoriasis, 89, 141, 147
Psorinum, 141
psychoneurosis, hypoglycaemic,
　84, 85
psychotherapy, 149
Pulsatilla, 23, 38, 40, 51, 110,
　112, 113, 115, 121, 149
Pyrogen, 30, 33, 52

quinsy, 40

reference, works of, 53-57
relapse, 68, 132-134
Relationship of Remedies, 45,
　129, 154
remedies, absorption of, 15, 19
　administration of, and storage,
　　15-17
　antidotal relationship of, 45
　antimiasmatic, 109, 125, 133-
　　135, 138-144
　common, in acute prescribing,
　　24, 25
　concept of, 11, 21
　constitutional, 75, 76, 103-108
　deep-acting, 109
　general constitutional, 109-
　　115, 125, 126
　general constitutional, mode of
　　administration, 127-135
　inimical relationship of, 45
　major general constitutional,
　　116-123
　pathological, 103-108, 125,
　　126, 128, 129, 132-135,
　　145-151
　peculiar taste of, 15

prepared from allergens,151
psycho-organotropic, 148-150
relationship of, 56, 57
shelf-life of, 17
remission, apparent, 61
repertory, 53-6, 113, 114
Repertory of Homoeopathic
　Materia Medica, 55
Rescue Remedy (Bach), 31, 47
Rhus toxicodendron, 40, 48, 49,
　103, 146, 147
Rhus venenata, 147
rubella, see German measles
rubric, 54
Ruta, 49

Sabadilla, 152, 153
sac. lac., 129
salt, 69, 70, 78
salts, tissue, 148
salt-substitute, 78
scarlet fever, 40
scars, 100
Schussler, Dr W.H., 148
sciatica, 49
scoliosis, 142
sea-sickness, 42, 43
Sepia, 121, 122, 147
sexes, different remedial
　sensitivities of, 110
shock, 31, 47
sickness, morning, 51
Silicea, 11, 45, 48, 122, 143, 148
Similia similibus curentur, 9, 54
similimum, 22, 24, 33, 55, 115,
　116
skin, infective disease of, 48, 66
skullcap, 101
Spongia tosta, 38
sprain, acute, 18, 19
sprain, recurrent, 142
steam, 36, 38
sting, insect, 31, 53
substances, pharmacologically
　inert crude, preparation of, 13
succussion, 11
sugar, 77
Sulphur, 23, 34, 39, 66, 76, 90,
　110, 111, 113, 122-124, 139-
　141, 153
sunstroke, 30
supplements, dietetic, 99-101
suppression, 33, 66, 103, 139
Sycosis, 142
Sycotic Co., 147
Symphoricarpus racemosus, 51
Symphytum, 49
symptoms, concomitant, 26, 146,
　147
　keynote, 116
　local, 26
　mental, 112
　'new', 134, 135
　peculiar (characteristic), 55,
　　113, 116
　residual, 134

syndrome, premenstrual, 86, 99,
　100, 147
Reiter's, 147
Synoptic Key of the Materia
　Medica, A, 55
syphilis, 65

Tarentula cubensis, 48, 153
teas, herbal, 101
teething, 30
tests, food allergy, 93, 94
therapy, modification of
　remedial, 132-135
threshold, allergic, 97, 98
thrush, 39
Thuja occidentalis, 67, 142
Thyroidinum, 147
tincture, mother (∅), 11, 15, 16,
　19
toenail, ingrowing, 48
tonsillitis, acute, 21, 22, 35, 40,
　44
totality, 27, 114
toxins, 104
tracheitis, acute, 37, 38
treatment, topical, 16, 18, 19
trepidation, 43
trial, clinical, 114
trigger-effect, 16, 18
trituration, 11
Tuberculinum, 65, 66, 125, 143,
　153
tuberculosis, 65, 66
typology, susceptible, 54, 115,
　116

ulcer, peptic, 81
ulceration, varicose, 100
Urtica urens, 16, 31
urticaria, 92, 93
usage, clinical, 114

vaccination, 67
Vaccinosis, 67, 142
Varicella, 42
veganism, 89
vegetables, 78, 79
vegetarianism, 89
veins, varicose, 100
Vitamin A, 100
Vitamin B group, 69, 100
Vitamin B6, 100
Vitamin B12, 70, 89
Vitamin C, 37, 69, 101, 152, 153
Vitamin D, 100
Vitamin E, 31, 100

warts, 142
whooping cough, 40, 42
wounds, 16, 18
wrist, sprained, 49
wry-neck, acute, 49

yeast, brewer's, 51, 71, 100
yoga, 85
yogurt, 39

zinc, 69, 100